Lyme Disease, Ticks

and

You

**A Guide to Navigating
Tick Bites, Lyme Disease and
Other Tick-Borne Infections**

Shelley Ball, PhD

FIREFLY BOOKS

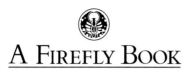

A FIREFLY BOOK

Published by Firefly Books Ltd. 2021
Copyright © 2021 Firefly Books Ltd.
Text © 2021 Shelley Ball
Photographs © as listed on page 160

First printing

Library of Congress Control Number: 2021932132

Library and Archives Canada Cataloguing in Publication
Title: Lyme disease, ticks and you : a guide to navigating tick bites, Lyme disease and other tick-borne infections / Shelley Ball, PhD.
Names: Ball, Shelley L. (Shelley Lynne), 1965- author.
Description: Includes bibliographical references.
Identifiers: Canadiana 20210129611 | ISBN 9780228103202 (softcover)
Subjects: LCSH: Lyme disease—Popular works. | LCSH: Tick-borne diseases—Popular works.
Classification: LCC RC155.5 .B35 2021 | DDC 616.9/246—dc23

Published in the United States by
Firefly Books (U.S.) Inc.
P.O. Box 1338, Ellicott Station
Buffalo, New York 14205

Published in Canada by
Firefly Books Ltd.
50 Staples Avenue, Unit 1
Richmond Hill, Ontario L4B 0A7

Editor: Julie Takasaki
Cover and interior design: Hartley Millson
Copyeditor: Anne Godlewski
Illustrations on pages 25, 28, 41, 46, 62, 65 and 118 by George A. Walker
Illustration on page 37 by Hartley Millson

Printed in Canada

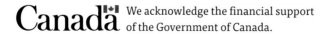

We acknowledge the financial support of the Government of Canada.

To those with Lyme disease and other tick-borne infections who suffer in silence and isolation. Don't give up! We *will* change things for the better.

CONTENTS

CHAPTER 5

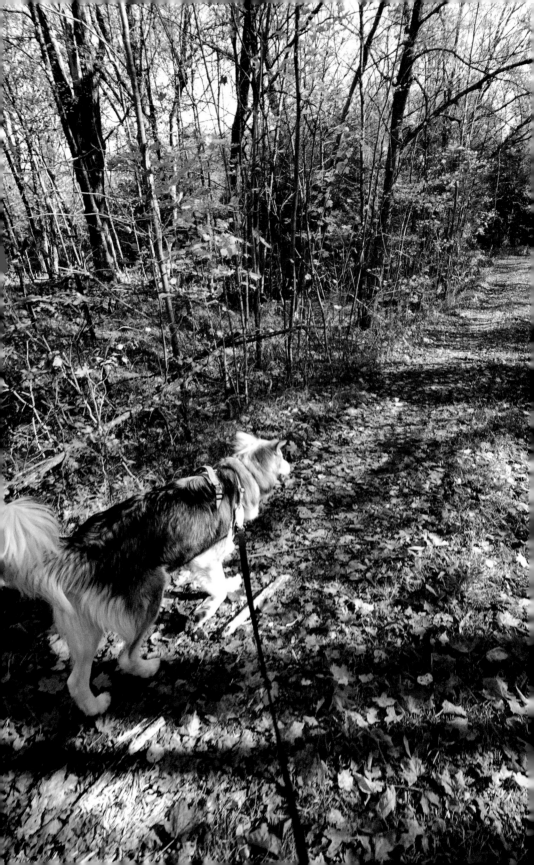

My Journey with Lyme Disease

When I found an engorged tick on my back in 2019, little did I know this discovery would lead to months of debilitating symptoms, dismissive arguments with many doctors, hours of research on Lyme and other tick-borne diseases (OTBDs) and effectively being abandoned by my public health care system.

Until recently, ticks weren't something I thought about. I've spent a great deal of my life outdoors: most of my childhood was spent outside, and in my work as an ecologist, I did a lot of field research. I had never even seen a tick until I participated in a two-month ecology program in Costa Rica while completing my PhD. I remember using duct tape to remove dozens of seed (larval) ticks after I happened to brush against a leaf on which many tiny ticks were perched, waiting for a mammal to walk by. I also pulled a fully engorged tick off my thigh after spending several days exploring a tropical forest. Back then it never dawned on me that these tiny arachnids could be carrying some microbe that could make me so sick. I was more worried about typhoid, malaria, dysentery, hepatitis or becoming a jaguar's dinner than I was about tick-borne diseases.

◀ My dog and I out for a walk in the woods near my home. My area is known as a Lyme disease hot spot in Ontario, Canada.

Fast forward a couple of decades to spring 2019. For the previous few years, I had been experiencing what I thought was burnout — feeling tired, listless and needing a break. Life was hectic with my job, volunteering and running an environmental organization from my home, and the years prior were filled with a series of life crises, including the illness and death of both my parents, a divorce and the temporary loss of my eyesight to cataracts. Surely stress and age eventually catch up with you, I thought, and you simply don't have the energy you did before.

When I found that fully engorged tick on my back, I knew I had to act right away. I live on 15 acres (6 hectares) of forest in what is considered a Lyme hotspot in Ontario, Canada. I understood that the longer the tick stayed on me, the greater the likelihood that it would transmit *Borrelia burgdorferi*, one of the bacteria that causes Lyme disease. Anxious to have it removed, I headed to the hospital.

The attending emergency room (ER) doctor removed the tick and prescribed two 200-milligram tablets of the antibiotic doxycycline. He assured me that if the tick was carrying Lyme bacteria, this single dose would kill them all. I was relieved to hear that. I asked if they could test the tick directly for the presence of the bacterium, but the attending nurse said no. (Though I didn't know this at the time, there are labs in Canada and the United States where you can get your tick tested. See page 76.) Nevertheless, I left the ER that day feeling safe with the knowledge that this dose of antibiotics the doctor gave me would keep me healthy.

And then the nightmare began.

Three days after my tick bite, I suddenly had sweats, followed by chills and aches, and I sensed a bad headache developing. I thought perhaps it was just the flu. After all, it was April and flu season wasn't over yet. I had these symptoms for several days, but about a week later I started to feel a bit better. Then I got hit with a cold, then an intense bout of seasonal allergies, and just as I was recovering, the body aches and other flu-like symptoms came back with a vengeance, along with full-body joint pain as I had never experienced before. The symptoms lessened after a couple of days and then returned again — even worse this time. Finally, out of desperation, I booked an appointment with my family doctor.

My doctor didn't think that Lyme was the cause, but she decided to run a blood test for it, along with tests for rheumatoid arthritis and several other diseases. She said a confirmatory Lyme test would be done again in a month in case I had Lyme but had not built up enough antibodies yet for the initial test to detect it.

My initial Lyme test came back negative, as did the confirmatory test and all the other tests she ran. By this point, I was only getting sicker, with new symptoms that included alternating chills and sweats at night and difficulty breathing. At times I felt as if I had an elephant sitting on my chest, as if my lungs wouldn't expand fully and I couldn't get a full breath.

A friend of mine who had been recovering from three tick-borne diseases suggested that my new symptoms sounded a lot like babesiosis. *Babesia* is a tick-borne blood parasite that, like the parasite that causes malaria, destroys red blood cells and can cause anemia and air hunger (an unexplained shortness of breath), among other symptoms. It sounded as if this could be the problem, so I got busy researching babesiosis, Lyme and OTBDs, going straight for the peer-reviewed papers published in reputable science journals. I wanted credible information on Lyme and the other diseases, not the popular press articles, although I did find the personal accounts in the press articles both fascinating and disturbing — especially the parts about the struggles of receiving a diagnosis and accessing treatment. It was because of reading these personal accounts and having ruled out other possible causes of my symptoms that I began to realize that everything I was experiencing pointed to Lyme disease and babesiosis.

My symptoms continued to get worse and worse, so I returned to my family doctor in late June, this time equipped with my research. My doctor said I couldn't be sick with Lyme disease because both my Lyme tests had come back negative and I had never presented with a bull's-eye rash — what is thought by many medical practitioners as the hallmark symptom of Lyme. My research showed that serologic (blood) tests are notoriously unreliable for diagnosing Lyme, and the bull's-eye rash appears not nearly as frequently as we have been led to believe. I insisted that a clinical diagnosis, which is based on symptoms and other factors, such as the patient's history, activity and location, is crucial when it comes to Lyme disease. After considerable discussion, she began to acknowledge that perhaps I was fighting a Lyme infection. She put me on three weeks of doxycycline, though she still wanted to test for lupus and other conditions.

As for the air hunger and alternating sweats and chills I was experiencing, my doctor didn't believe I had babesiosis because my tests showed I was not anemic. This puzzled me — I presented other symptoms of the disease, so doesn't it make sense to treat for babesiosis before I develop signs of anemia?

Desperate for more help, I booked an appointment with a naturopath who was recommended by a friend. My friend's husband had been diagnosed with Lyme disease after being ill for several years, and he had really benefited from naturopathic treatment. I have to admit, I was initially skeptical that a naturopath could help, but as a scientist I also knew that many naturopathic remedies are effective because they contain compounds, most often isolated from plants, that have medicinal effects. Many of these compounds are the basis for synthetic drugs. My first appointment involved a thorough discussion not just about my symptoms, but also about the history of those symptoms. I mentioned feeling burned out for the past few years. She asked whether I had been bitten by a tick previously, and although I recalled finding a raised bite mark on my neck in fall 2017, I had not actually seen a tick. I had tested negative for Lyme disease then. I also recalled finding a small, red, raised oval-shaped rash on my leg in 2015. I initially thought it was a spider bite; it certainly didn't look like the bull's-eye rash that I had heard was associated with Lyme disease. That's when the naturopath showed me photos of other Lyme rashes. My 2015 rash looked very similar to some of those examples.

Her clinical diagnosis was that I not only had babesiosis (and possibly bartonellosis, another tick-borne disease caused by *Bartonella* bacteria), but that I had likely contracted Lyme disease a few years before then, if not earlier, and had been dealing with a low-level infection for a while. Because I was no longer dealing with an acute case of Lyme disease, the naturopath said I needed another three weeks of antibiotics. I contacted my family doctor and shared the results of my consultation with the naturopath. She was hesitant to prescribe the additional three weeks of doxycycline; however, after more discussion she finally gave me the prescription. I felt privileged to have been given the longer course of antibiotics, and I attributed it to my in-depth research into Lyme literature. For most patients, receiving additional treatment is a rarity.

While on the antibiotics, I felt better than I had in years. My energy improved, the joint pain was lessening and the night sweats, chills and air hunger were slowly decreasing. It was like the light at the end of the tunnel. However, after the antibiotics ended in early August, I started to feel unwell again. It wasn't one specific symptom, but rather I started to feel progressively lousier until I was sicker than I was before I had started the antibiotics. Concerned about my extreme fatigue and air hunger, my family doctor checked my blood oxygen levels and ordered an electrocardiogram (ECG), a spirometry test, a chest X-ray, a cardiac stress test, an echocardiogram and more blood tests. Everything came back normal. She was disturbed at my condition and yet nothing abnormal was showing in any test results. She referred me to an infectious disease doctor, but the doctor refused to see me after I mentioned Lyme disease. This was disturbing to me. No doctor should refuse a patient because of the diseases they have or think they have.

As the month wore on, I was less able to function day-to-day: my Lyme, bartonellosis and babesiosis symptoms were so bad that I couldn't even climb the 13 steps to my home office upstairs. To be honest, I felt as though I was dying. I ended up at the ER one weekend because I couldn't breathe, my joints ached so terribly that I could hardly get out of bed, my short-term memory was lapsing, I was having trouble speaking and remembering words and I had no energy, a persistent headache, swollen glands and constant ear ringing.

My experience in the ER of my local hospital was not a good one. I explained the progression of my symptoms to the attending doctor, but as soon as I said the words "Lyme disease," the doctor seemed to check out of our discussion and even became belliger-ent when I disagreed with him about his views on Lyme. He could see I was clearly very sick and completely at my wit's end. He ordered several tests to rule out anything of immediate concern, and all of my results came back normal. I explained to him that I had done my research and knew that we should expect these various tests to be normal with Lyme disease as the culprit, and he replied that there was not much more he could do for me. He offered to submit a request for a consultation with a local internal medicine doctor, but this consultation never happened. When I called to book an appointment, as soon as I mentioned Lyme, I was told that the internal medicine doctor would not see me.

This was my introduction to being essentially abandoned by my public health care system because of my Lyme disease. Without a bull's-eye rash or a positive serologic test, no doctor would prescribe any treatment for me beyond what my family doctor had already given — or take the diagnosis of Lyme disease seriously, for that matter. I continued to get sicker and sicker. In addition to all my recurring symptoms, I also started experiencing neurological issues. My short-term memory was shot, I could barely read five sentences, I was forgetting the names of people I knew and I often couldn't think of the word I needed when speaking. It became even more frightening when I began to experience numbness around my mouth and on the left side of my face, tingling in my arms and fingers and such intense pressure on the left side of my head that I felt as though my brain would ooze out through my ear. I went back to my family doctor for help. She was shocked at my deterioration and told me to go back to the ER.

A different attending doctor *once again* told me I couldn't possibly have Lyme disease, and I *once again* recited my research. I also mentioned babesiosis. When the doctor realized I had done my homework and knew enough about Lyme and OTBDs, he began to take me more seriously. He did think my symptoms were characteristic of babesiosis, which was surprising to me since most family and ER doctors have never even heard of it. He ran an ECG to check my heart, took chest X-rays, did a urine analysis and drew 14 vials of blood along with enough blood for three blood culture bottles. The only abnormal result was that my white blood cell count was elevated, indicating I was fighting some sort of infection. The doctor referred me to the hospital's infectious disease doctor (the same one my family doctor had referred me to a month earlier) and then sent me home — no medication, no treatment, no help. The ER doctor had asked the infectious disease doctor to book an appointment with me as soon as possible. I didn't hear from that infectious disease doctor's office for another two months, and I finally saw another infectious disease doctor from the same clinic nearly five months after the initial referral.

Feeling utterly cast aside with no path forward, I joined a Lyme Facebook group and started begging for help. I talked to people who were either battling Lyme or knew someone who was. From these conversations, it seemed I had three options:

1. Go to British Columbia to be seen by a naturopathic doctor who could prescribe antibiotics (it is the only province in Canada where a naturopath can prescribe them).
2. Go to the United States to be seen by a Lyme-literate medical doctor.
3. Try to get an appointment with a Lyme-literate medical doctor at a private clinic in Ontario.

All of these options meant I would have to pay for treatment out of my own pocket. Eventually, I chose option 3. I waited two excruciating months for an appointment, but I can't tell you the sense of relief I felt when I finally got to speak with a medical practitioner who understood what I was going through and who had the science and medical expertise to help me.

I was diagnosed with chronic (sometimes referred to as "per-sister") Lyme disease, babesiosis, bartonellosis and a mold infection. Sadly, coinfections with *Babesia* and *Bartonella* are common among people with chronic Lyme disease, and they make it much harder to eradicate the illness. As well, mold infections, which are picked up from various molds that live in the environment, suppress the immune system and often open the door for Lyme to take hold. Until proper immune function is restored, reducing or eradicating Lyme and OTBDs can be challenging, if not impossible. My current treatment for chronic Lyme focuses on restoring my immune function, reducing the rampant systemic inflammation that had taken over my body, and killing the *Borrelia, Babesia, Bartonella* and mold infections. Killing needs to be done in stages, and some treatments aren't even worth attempting until immune function is restored. This is why recovering from Lyme and OTBDs can be a long, drawn-out process — a marathon, not a sprint.

As of writing this book I continue to receive treatment from a private clinic run by doctors who are experts on Lyme and OTBDs. Although I am still battling my infections (including new Lyme

What Is a Lyme-Literate Doctor?

Lyme-literate doctors specialize in tick-borne illnesses and typically immerse themselves in the peer-reviewed science of Lyme and OTBDs. They regularly attend conferences and communicate with peers who also specialize in tick-borne illnesses so they can stay current on research and new treatment options.

and *Babesia* infections from 2020), my treatments have helped me enormously. I experience flare-ups, which can be pretty rough and make me feel as if I'm right back to square one, but for the most part, I feel pretty good — certainly better than I have been feeling for the past four years. My diagnosis and treatment have so far cost me over $25,000 because they are not covered by any of my health plans. I pay over $1,000 per month for ongoing treatment, which will likely continue well into the future. Unfortunately, if you have chronic Lyme, as I do, you must be prepared to pay a lot of money out of your own pocket for treatment and accept that it could take months to years to be cured, if ever.

Hindsight is 20/20. With what I have experienced and learned about Lyme disease and OTBDs, as well as mold infections, I can now look back and put together the pieces of my puzzling journey with Lyme disease.

I realize now that I was likely infected with Lyme years ago, if not decades. It was in 2016 that I really started to experience feeling run-down and depressed, and I thought it was just the culmination of years of stress from overworking and significant life crises. And I'm sure it was, in part. It was likely the prolonged stress that caused my immune system to become compromised, opening the door for the mold, Lyme and other tick-borne infections to take hold.

I also realize now that the solid, raised rash I found on my leg in the summer of 2015 was likely a result of being bitten by a

Borrelia-carrying tick. As I will discuss in more depth later, not all people infected with Lyme exhibit a rash. In fact, as few as 9 percent of those infected exhibit the bull's-eye rash (Stonehouse et al. 2010), and there is now evidence showing that the Lyme rash is highly variable. Had I known this back in 2015, I may have been able to avoid the nightmare that I am dealing with today.

This is one of many reasons it is critical to understand the current scientific literature about Lyme disease and OTBDs. Unfortunately, so much information shared by public health units is out of date and does not reflect the current peer-reviewed science, meaning most of our medical practitioners will be of little help when dealing with a possible Lyme or OTBD diagnosis.

All of this leads me to the reason I have written this book and why I am sharing my story with you. My experience is not unique. In fact, it is far too common. The number of people I have connected with who have similar stories is both frightening and discouraging. The level of abandonment by medical systems that Lyme sufferers feel is concerning. Through this book I want to help you understand Lyme disease, reduce your chances of a tick bite, determine whether you have contracted Lyme (or another tick-borne disease) and, if you do have Lyme disease or an OTBD, find help in nontraditional places.

In writing this book, I thought to myself, What do I wish I had known when I found that fully engorged tick in 2019? What information would have helped me understand my symptoms and obtain a diagnosis and treatment faster? Because many public health systems offer little to no help for those with Lyme, especially for those who test negative or do not present a bull's-eye rash, I want to help people become strong self-advocates who can fight for the health care they need. Sadly, the only way you will get help is by becoming a well-informed and vocal self-advocate.

A number of excellent and detailed books have been published about Lyme disease (and OTBDs) and its diagnosis and treatment. I have listed some of these in the Resources section of this book and encourage you to consult them if you want more details than I present here. These books contain a wealth of information, but many have so much detail that the average person may struggle to understand everything. My goal with this book is to take the key information from such detailed books, the peer-reviewed published science articles and the websites of reputable advocacy groups and distill everything down in a way that anyone can grasp. Without knowledge of the basic information as well as the misinformation surrounding Lyme disease and OTBDs, it is challenging, if not impossible, to self-advocate for diagnosis and treatment.

If Lyme disease (and OTBDs) is already an issue in your life, then I hope this book helps you navigate the complex and challenging journey you are on. I have included a collection of resources at the back of this book, including peer-reviewed science articles, books, websites, videos and podcasts.

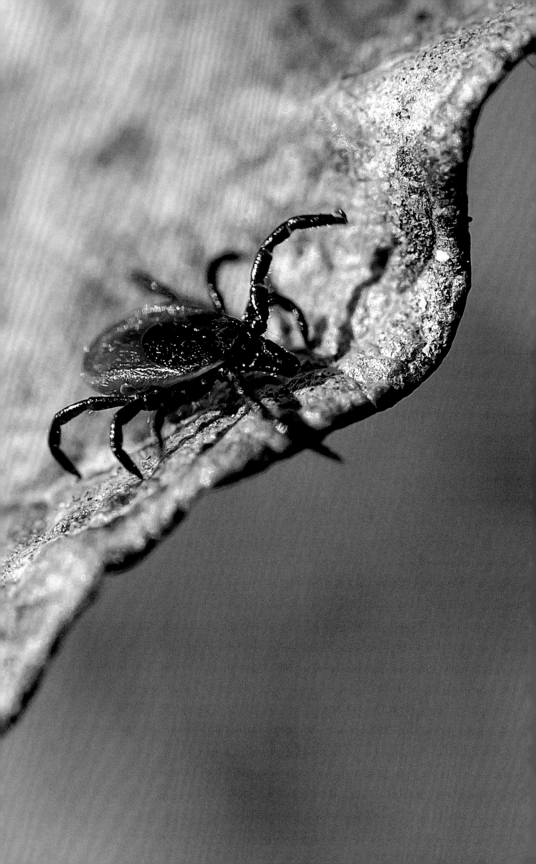

CHAPTER **1**

What You Need to Know About Ticks and Lyme Disease

WHAT IS LYME DISEASE?

Lyme disease is a bacterial infection that is spread through the bite of an infected tick. The primary species of bacteria that causes Lyme in North America is *Borrelia burgdorferi*, although we now know that other *Borrelia* species and strains also cause Lyme and Lyme-like diseases, including relapsing fever. The *Borrelia* bacterium is a spirochete, which means it is corkscrew-shaped. The corkscrew shape helps the bacterium persist in the human body because it can bore into tissues and "hide" after the acute infection phase is over. The shape of the bacterium can also change during its life cycle, which allows it to form a dormant,

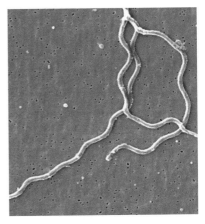

A scanning electron microscope image of *Borrelia burgdorferi*, a species of bacteria that causes Lyme disease.

◀ Ticks enjoy moist conditions and are typically found in leaf litter.

cystic round body that can evade most antibiotic treatment and persist in the body for months or years (Sapi et al. 2019).

In later chapters I will delve deeper into how Lyme bacteria infect the body, often persevering even after antibiotics have been taken, as well as why the bacteria make us sick.

A Brief History of Lyme Disease

B. burgdorferi has been around for a long time. Due to the increased prevalence of Lyme disease globally, it is only recently that the disease has received a lot of attention. *Borrelia* species have been found in ticks trapped inside pieces of amber that date back 15 to 20 million years (Poinar 2015). In terms of evidence of human infection, a forensic genetic study of ancient human remains that date back 5,300 years and were recovered from a glacier in the Italian Alps revealed the presence of *B. burgdorferi* (Keller et al. 2012).

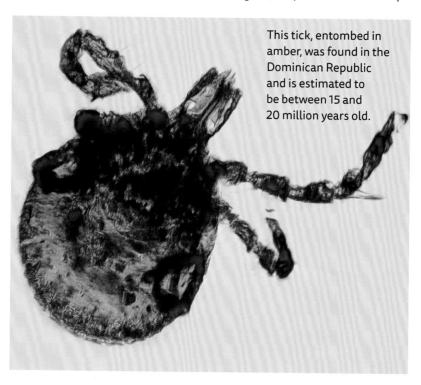

This tick, entombed in amber, was found in the Dominican Republic and is estimated to be between 15 and 20 million years old.

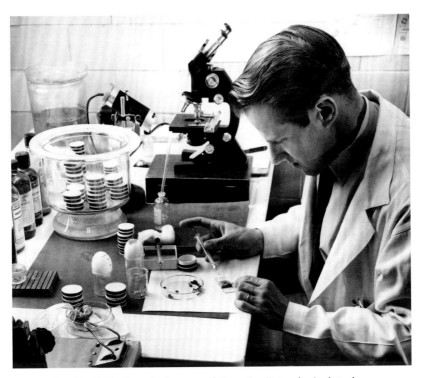

A portrait of Dr. Willy Burgdorfer, one of the scientists who isolated
B. burgdorferi.

While Lyme disease is not new, the medical profession did not
really know about it until the mid-1970s. It was only then that
Lyme officially became a diagnosable disease.

In November 1975, a mysterious illness hit the town of Lyme,
Connecticut. Fifty-one people (39 children and 12 adults) suddenly
and simultaneously became ill. The one thing common to all of
these people was that they had been bitten by ticks (Edlow 2003).
Initially the illness was thought to be a viral infection, but ground-
breaking work by Dr. Willy Burgdorfer and his colleagues at the
Rocky Mountain Laboratories of the National Institute of Allergy
and Infectious Diseases led to the isolation of a corkscrew-like bacterium in the blood of these patients. This new-to-medical-science
bacterium was named *"Borrelia burgdorferi"* in honor of Dr.

Burgdorfer, its discoverer. Although Dr. Burgdorfer and his colleagues were the first to isolate the bacterium and determine that it was responsible for what we now call Lyme disease, accounts of cases of an illness with the same symptoms had been described in Europe and North America for over a hundred years. The bull's-eye rash (also called *erythema migrans* or the EM rash) had been noted by physicians earlier in the 20th century, but no official name was given to the disease until Dr. Burgdorfer's discovery.

WHY ARE WE SEEING A SURGE?

In North America, we have been hearing much more about Lyme disease in the past five to 10 years. If the disease has been afflicting humans for thousands of years, why then has Lyme become a hot topic so recently? The incidence of Lyme disease is on the rise globally. In North America, Lyme disease is the most prevalent vector-borne disease, which is defined as a disease caused by a microorganism and transmitted by an animal. The Centers for Disease Control and Prevention (CDC) in the United States estimate there are as many as 300,000 cases of Lyme disease in the United States annually. The numbers in Canada are significantly lower, with the Public Health Agency of Canada (PHAC) reporting just 1,487 cases in 2018. However, researchers believe this is a gross underestimation, which is a result of Canada's case definition of Lyme disease, its underreporting of clinically diagnosed acute cases and its overreliance on inadequate serologic testing (Lloyd and Hawkins 2018).

Climate change is cited as one of the main factors for the increased incidence of tick bites and tick-borne diseases globally (Pfeiffer 2018). As our climate has warmed, black-legged ticks, the ticks that carry *Borrelia* and other microbes (such as bacteria, viruses and protozoans), have expanded their range in North America. These two maps on the right show how the range of the black-legged tick in the U.S., particularly in the northeast and upper Midwest, has increased significantly between 1996 and 2020.

U.S. distribution of black-legged ticks in 1996

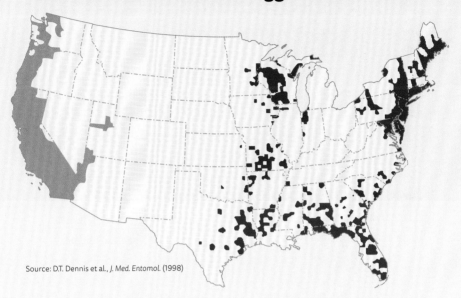

Source: D.T. Dennis et al., *J. Med. Entomol.* (1998)

U.S. distribution of black-legged ticks in 2020

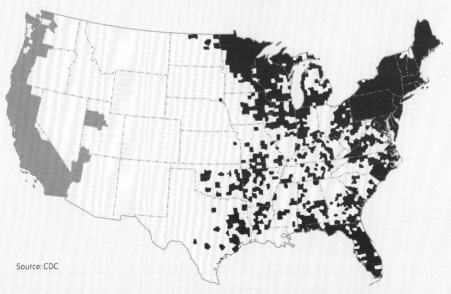

Source: CDC

Areas where *Ixodes pacificus* established populations have been documented.

Areas where *Ixodes scapularis* established populations have been documented.

This means that these ticks are moving into areas where they had not previously been abundant. Ticks love heat and humidity, so as our planet heats up and parts of the world become warmer and wetter, more tick-friendly conditions are being created. In eastern North America, milder and wetter winters mean that ticks can safely overwinter, whereas many of them would have been killed in the colder winters of the past. So, not only is the tick expanding its range, its population is also growing.

Human encounters with tick habitats are increasing as well. Certainly in the United States and Canada there is a trend toward building new housing developments on the city outskirts, on former farmland or in forested areas. As urban sprawl continues and more people spend time in the kinds of habitats where ticks thrive (tall grasses, shrubby areas and forests), the likelihood of tick bites increases. And as more people get out to enjoy outdoor activities such as hiking and camping, the likelihood of encountering ticks goes up. Are these reasons enough to live only in the city or to stop enjoying nature? Absolutely not! I can't emphasize enough how these are not reasonable solutions, especially when a number of studies show the health and well-being benefits of spending time in nature. Instead of avoiding the outdoors, we should all be taking precautions to reduce the likelihood of a tick bite, and there are simple, common-sense measures that can be taken. (For tips, see Chapter 3.)

Several other factors are thought to be at play with the increased frequency of tick bites and incidence of Lyme disease. One of the primary hosts of Lyme bacteria is mice, particularly the white-footed mouse (*Peromyscus leucopus*). Mouse populations are on the rise due to human impacts, and urban sprawl has brought more humans to places where mice naturally occur. Climate change may be creating more favorable conditions for mouse and small rodent (squirrels, chipmunks, etc.) populations, leading to increased population sizes. As an example, my own backyard,

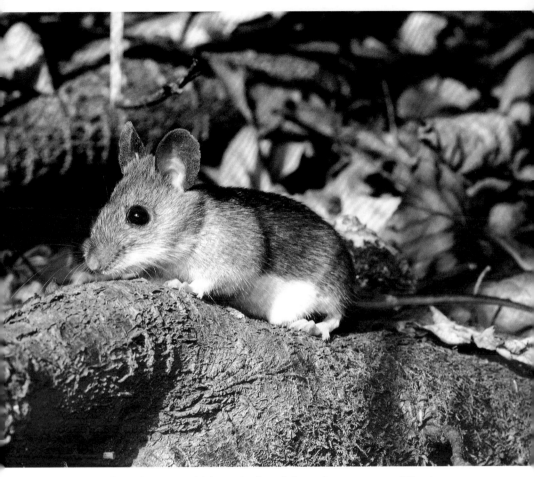

The white-footed mouse, which can be found through many parts of North America, is one of the primary hosts of *B. burgdorferi*.

which consists mostly of mixed coniferous-deciduous forest, contains a number of oak trees. With oak trees come acorns, and in 2015 the oak trees produced a bumper crop of acorns. In the few years that followed, the small-rodent population seemed to explode, and with that came ticks. Before 2015, I had never encountered a tick in my backyard, but now, in spring and fall, I can't spend five minutes in my backyard without finding one crawling on me.

North American Migratory Bird Flyways

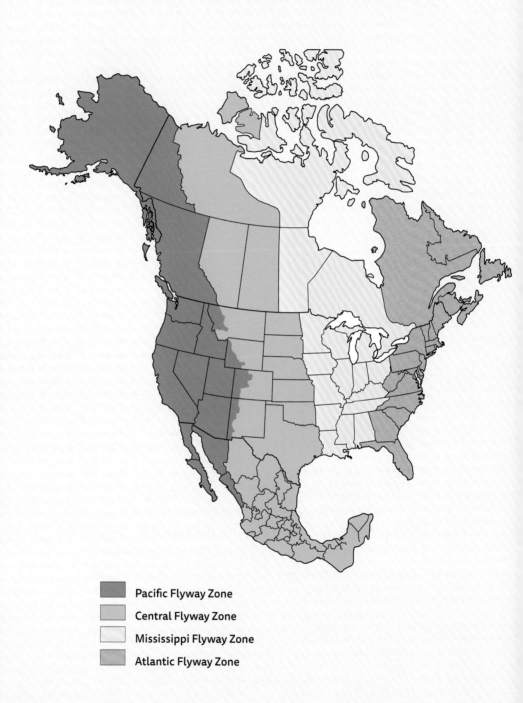

■ Pacific Flyway Zone
■ Central Flyway Zone
□ Mississippi Flyway Zone
■ Atlantic Flyway Zone

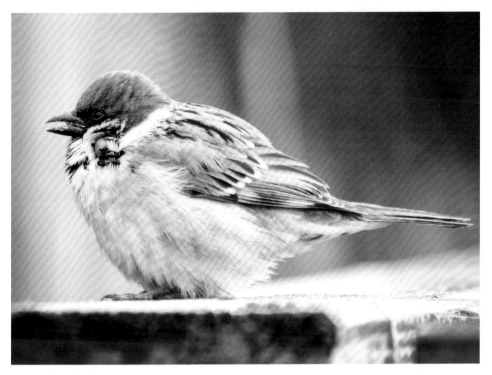

This bird is carrying an engorged tick on its neck.

The prevalence of Lyme disease is also related to the movement of migratory birds (Anderson et al. 1986; Scott and Durden 2015). The map shown here illustrates the main flyways migratory birds in North America use.

Ticks attach to and feed on birds, so each spring, as birds migrate north for the summer, some birds can bring ticks with them. Once a tick is done feeding, it unlatches itself from its bird host and falls to the ground, only to wait to latch onto another host when it is ready to feed again. These ticks might be carrying strains of *Borrelia* bacteria (or other microbes) that typically occur farther south. Does this mean that migratory birds are responsible for the rise in tick bites and Lyme disease? No. There is little doubt that birds have been transporting ticks north for a very long time. However, because climate change is creating more favorable conditions for ticks in winter, those ticks that do hitchhike north are less likely to be killed by colder weather. As you can see, it is the combined effects of several factors, not just one, that are responsible for the explosion of tick populations and, consequently, the increased incidence of Lyme and other tick-borne diseases (OTBDs) in more northerly locations.

Don't look at our migratory birds as a source of fear. I have heard accounts of individuals and even organizations advocating for removing bird feeders to reduce tick populations. In my view, this is misguided advice. A few birds in your backyard are unlikely to lead to a massive tick infestation, and ticks can just as easily drop from flying birds or birds that happen to land in your yard even if you don't have a feeder. Our songbirds are in peril, and bird feeders help to sustain their populations. Rather than discouraging birds, feel free to feed and enjoy watching them, but take simple precautions to minimize your risk of encountering a tick.

It is important to recognize that the increased incidence of Lyme may also be due to heightened awareness of the disease, which would lead to more frequent diagnoses than in the past. There are now more Lyme-literate doctors, particularly in the United States, who understand the science of Lyme disease; however, there are still significant challenges in getting doctors in the United States and, especially, Canada to rely on a clinical diagnosis of Lyme based on symptoms and history rather than depending too heavily on unreliable serologic tests. In Canada, without a bull's-eye rash or a positive Lyme test, you are unlikely to be offered treatment for Lyme disease, despite your symptoms.

Far too often, doctors dismiss the possibility of Lyme disease. I have heard and read about many instances in the United States and Canada of a person having Lyme disease for years, sometimes decades, and that the disease went undetected because their doctor never suspected it or refused to consider Lyme disease as a possible diagnosis. Lyme disease is often referred to as "the great imitator" because so many of the symptoms are also common to other medical conditions, and a clinical diagnosis of Lyme is easy to overlook if a doctor does not know to look for it. This is why it is critical for doctors to know the current scientific literature on Lyme disease and understand how to diagnose it clinically.

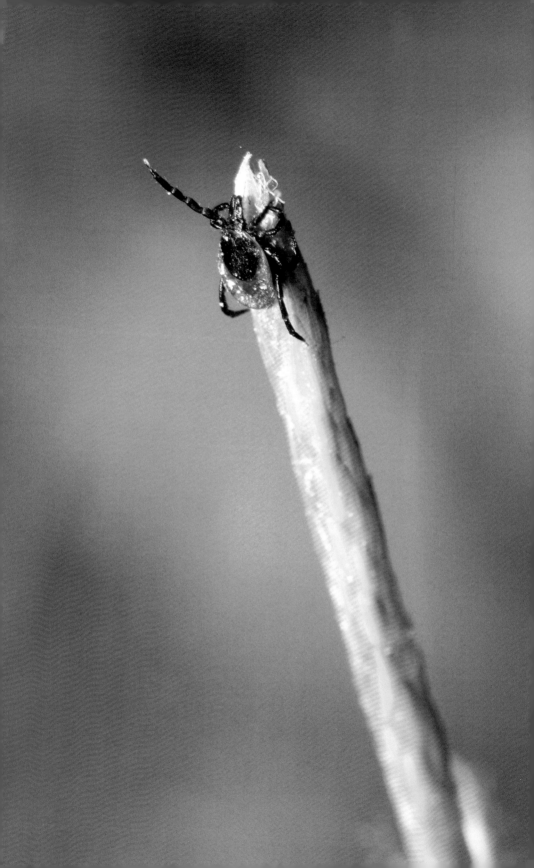

CHAPTER **2**

The Biology of Lyme Disease

TAXONOMY AND LYME DISEASE

What is taxonomy and why do you need to know about it when it comes to Lyme disease? Taxonomy refers to the science of naming organisms. It is a construct used to catalog biological diversity and give us labels that we can use to accurately identify individual species. The scientific name of an organism consists of two names, the first being the genus and the second being the species. The genus is always capitalized, and both names are styled in italics. For example, the main tick species that transmits Lyme disease in North America is

Ixodes scapularis

Ixodes is the genus name, and *scapularis* is the species name.

Common names (the nonscientific name given to an organism) can be problematic because different people might use the same common name to refer to different species. Or we can have the

◄ An *Ixodes* tick waits at the top of a stem for an animal to pass so it can latch on for a blood meal.

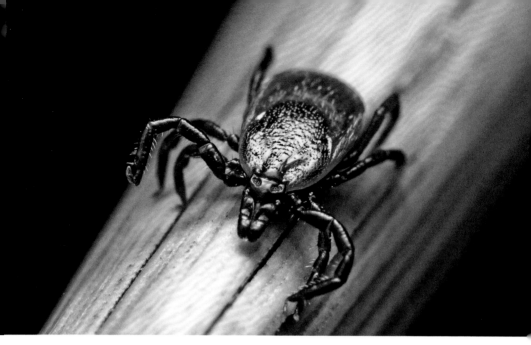

A black-legged tick (*Ixodes scapularis*), the main species of tick that transmits Lyme disease in North America.

opposite problem, where different common names are used to refer to the same species. For example, some people will call *Ixodes scapularis* a deer tick, while others will tell you it's a black-legged tick, but they are the same species. Using a scientific name can help avoid confusion and ensure we are referring to the same organism.

The Taxonomy of *Borrelia*

The species of bacteria that causes Lyme disease belongs to a *species complex* (Rudenko et al. 2011). This is a group of species in the same genus (in this case, *Borrelia*) that are very closely related genetically. When most physicians who are not Lyme experts (such as your family doctor or an ER doctor) refer to Lyme bacteria, they are typically referring to a specific species of bacteria called B. *burgdorferi sensu stricto* (*sensu stricto* means "in the strict sense" in Latin), which is the primary cause of Lyme disease in North America. B. *burgdorferi sensu lato* (*sensu lato* means "in the general sense") consists of a group of *Borrelia* species that are genetically very similar to B. *burgdorferi sensu stricto* and are associated with Lyme disease.

A Note on Naming

For ease of reading, when I am referring generally to the bacterium that causes Lyme disease in North America, I will simply call it B. burgdorferi, Borrelia bacteria or Lyme bacteria. I will add sl after the name B. burgdorferi when I need to refer to the species complex, and I will add ss after the name when I need to distinguish between the species complex and the species in the strict sense. When presenting information on other Borrelia species within the complex, I will use specific species names (for example, B. afzelii).

Worldwide, there are at least 52 species in the genus Borrelia (Cutler et al. 2017). There are 21 species in the B. burgdorferi sl species complex that are associated with Lyme disease; 29 are associated primarily with relapsing fevers (Binetruy et al. 2020). Within B. burgdorferi sl are a large number of strains. Strains show genetic differences, but those differences are too small to classify them as separate species. Scientists are far from understanding the significance of this genetic diversity. However, there is some evidence that suggests different strains may cause different Lyme disease symptoms, so understanding what species or strain has infected a person may become very important as we learn more about the biology of various strains (Stanek and Reiter 2011; Tijsse-Klassen et al. 2013).

You may wonder why you should care about the taxonomy of Borrelia. Understanding the taxonomy is particularly important in Lyme disease testing. For example, testing for B. burgdorferi ss when a patient is actually infected with B. afzelii, a European species, will usually yield a negative result. The patient may indeed be ill with Lyme disease, but if it wasn't caused by the Borrelia species that is typically tested for in North America, the test will likely fail to detect the Borrelia infection. As we will get into in Chapter 5, a Lyme test can be negative for a number of reasons, and it isn't simply because the person doesn't have the disease. This example also illustrates why we should care about what *Borrelia* species occur elsewhere in the world. *B. burgdorferi ss* is the main species that causes Lyme disease in North America, but the ease and extent of global travel mean that humans can be exposed to species that they wouldn't normally encounter. For example, there are three *Borrelia* species that are primarily responsible for cases of Lyme disease in Europe: *B. garinii*, *B. afzelii* and *B. burgdorferi ss*. If a person who has traveled in Europe presents symptoms of Lyme disease after they return home, their physician would need to run additional, separate tests specifically for the European species to detect possible infection by them, but this is not a standard approach that most doctors take.

THE LIFE CYCLES OF TICKS AND LYME BACTERIA

To understand the life cycle of *B. burgdorferi*, we need to understand the life cycle of its vector, the tick. In North America, it is the black-legged tick (also known as the deer tick) that is primarily responsible for the transmission of *B. burgdorferi*. There are two species of black-legged tick in North America, both belonging to the genus *Ixodes*: *Ixodes scapularis*, which is found in eastern and central North America; and *Ixodes pacificus*, which is found in western North America.

Ticks are not insects. Rather, they are arachnids — the group that contains spiders and mites. This means they have eight legs, whereas insects have six. The black-legged tick belongs to a group known as *hard ticks* (family Ixodidae). This refers to the fact that, as nymphs and adults, they have a hard exoskeleton (or external skeleton). In contrast, *soft ticks* (family Argasidae) are entirely soft-bodied.

Close to 100 species of hard ticks are found in North America, but aside from the two species of black-legged tick mentioned above, most are not known to transmit Lyme disease. There are,

Estimated Distribution of Black-Legged Ticks in Canada and the United States

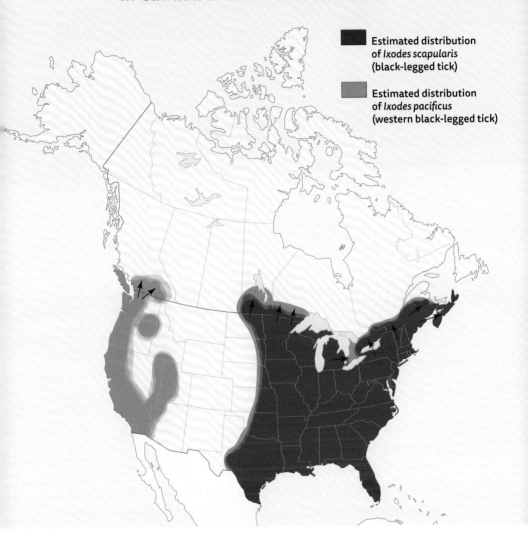

■ Estimated distribution of *Ixodes scapularis* (black-legged tick)

■ Estimated distribution of *Ixodes pacificus* (western black-legged tick)

however, species that transmit other diseases, as you can see on the table on pages 38–39. Black-legged ticks also transmit more than just Lyme bacteria. *Ixodes scapularis* can transmit the microbes that cause anaplasmosis, relapsing fever, ehrlichiosis, babesiosis, bartonellosis and Powassan virus. *Ixodes pacificus* can transmit bacteria that cause anaplasmosis and relapsing fever.

Common Disease-Transmitting Ticks

Tick	Scientific Name	Distribution	Diseases Transmitted
Black-legged tick * (also known as a deer tick) 	*Ixodes scapularis*	Widely distributed across the eastern United States and Canada	• Lyme disease (*B. burgdorferi*, *B. mayonii*) • Anaplasmosis • Babesiosis • Bartonellosis • Relapsing fever (*B. miyamotoi*) • Ehrlichiosis • Tick-borne meningoencephalitis • Powassan virus
Western black-legged tick * 	*Ixodes pacificus*	Along the Pacific coast of the U.S. and Canada, particularly northern California	• Lyme disease (*B. burgdorferi*) • Anaplasmosis • Relapsing fever (*B. miyamotoi*)
American dog tick * 	*Dermacentor variabilis*	Widely distributed east of the Rocky Mountains, and in limited areas on the Pacific coast of the U.S.	• Rocky Mountain spotted fever • Tularemia
Brown dog tick 	*Rhipicephalus sanguineus*	Across North America	• Rocky Mountain spotted fever

Tick	Scientific Name	Distribution	Diseases Transmitted
Lone star tick *	*Amblyomma americanum*	South-central, central and eastern U.S. and parts of Ontario and Quebec	• Ehrlichiosis • Southern tick-associated rash illness (STARI) • Heartland virus • Bourbon virus • Possible severe allergy to red meat
Pacific coast tick	*Dermacentor occidentalis*	Pacific coast of U.S. and Canada	• Rocky Mountain spotted fever • Colorado tick fever • Tularemia
Gulf coast tick	*Amblyomma maculatum*	Gulf of Mexico and mid-Atlantic coast	• Rickettsiosis
Rocky Mountain wood tick	*Dermacentor andersoni*	Rocky Mountain states and British Columbia, Alberta and Saskatchewan	• Rocky Mountain spotted fever • Tularemia • Colorado tick fever
Groundhog tick	*Ixodes cookei*	Eastern U.S., central and eastern Canada	• Powassan virus

* Ticks that commonly bite humans

To complete its life cycle, a tick needs to latch onto an animal to obtain a blood meal multiple times over its development. Typically, black-legged ticks will look for a mammal or bird to latch onto, but they are opportunists and are capable of feeding on reptiles and even amphibians. When a tick feeds on an animal that is carrying *Borrelia* bacteria, it becomes infected and, thus, a carrier of the bacteria and can infect any animals it subsequently feeds on, including humans.

Feeding on an animal host is critical for the survival and reproduction of both the tick and the bacteria. If it weren't for the tick seeking a blood meal from an animal, the Lyme bacteria would never make contact with new animal hosts. The tick and *Borrelia* bacteria have evolved in step together, reaching a kind of evolutionary truce. *Borrelia* depends on the tick to move it from host to host, but the tick itself does not become ill from its presence.

The life cycle of the black-legged tick generally takes two years to complete, although this may vary by geography. Ticks have four life stages: egg, larva, nymph and adult. A tick needs to feed repeatedly to complete its life cycle. It was generally thought that the black-legged tick needs three hosts over the course of its life; however, there is now evidence that ticks may actually feed more than this, sometimes having partial feedings and then dropping off their hosts before becoming fully engorged (Shih and Spielman 1993).

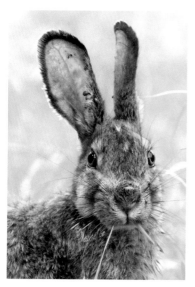

This wild rabbit's face and ears are covered in engorged ticks.

When an egg of a black-legged tick hatches, typically in late summer, the larva that emerges must have a blood meal to survive, and to grow and develop into a nymph, the next stage

The Life Cycle of a Black-Legged Tick

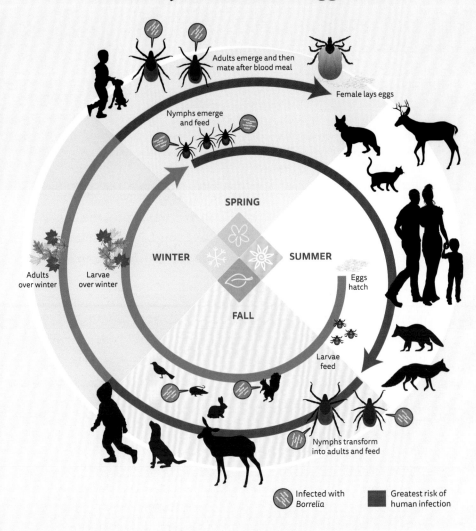

Adults emerge and then mate after blood meal

Female lays eggs

Nymphs emerge and feed

SPRING

WINTER

SUMMER

Adults over winter

Larvae over winter

Eggs hatch

FALL

Larvae feed

Nymphs transform into adults and feed

Infected with *Borrelia*

Greatest risk of human infection

in its development. The larva stays on the ground, waiting for a small animal host, such as a mouse, rabbit, chipmunk or squirrel, to brush past. The larva attaches itself to the host and begins feeding on its blood. Once it has fed sufficiently, it drops off and continues to grow until it molts and becomes a nymph. It's important to note that newly hatched larvae do not carry *Borrelia* bacteria. It is not until the larva bites an animal host already infected with

Location, Location, Location

Clearly, not all black-legged ticks are infected with *B. burgdorferi* or other species of disease-causing microbes. The incidence of infection varies geographically. Some places are hot spots, meaning they have a high incidence of *B. burgdorferi* (a large percentage of ticks test positive for the bacterium). For example, I live not far from an area in which 80 percent of the ticks sampled in one study were carrying *B. burgdorferi* (Clow 2017).

To find out where cases have been reported in your state or province, check with your local public health agency. Bear in mind that Lyme cases are notoriously underreported, and it's difficult for any public health agency to precisely define geographic limits on tick populations.

Borrelia bacteria that it is then infected and becomes a vector for Lyme disease.

The nymphs overwinter in leaf litter in forests and grassy (including your lawn) or shrubby areas. In the spring, the nymphs emerge, hungry for a blood meal and actively looking for a host to feed on. This is why spring is one of the riskiest times of year for tick bites; it's when ticks are hungry, and the environmental conditions are cool and wet — ideal for ticks. If the larva from the previous year fed on a host that was not carrying Lyme bacteria, its feeding the following spring presents another opportunity for it to become infected. Fall is also a risky time of year because ticks are looking for their last blood meal of the season, and the cooler weather also means a moister environment — something ticks like.

By the fall, the nymph matures into an adult, and once again it overwinters in leaf litter. Males and females emerge in very early spring and mate. Males will feed intermittently, while females must have a blood meal to produce eggs, so they will actively look for a host. Female black-legged ticks lay up to 3,000 eggs at a time, which hatch in late summer, beginning the next generation of ticks.

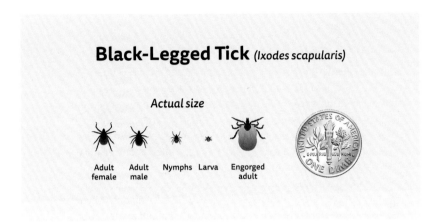

Black-Legged Tick *(Ixodes scapularis)*

Actual size

Adult female	Adult male	Nymphs	Larva	Engorged adult	

Larval black-legged ticks have six legs and are generally lighter colored. Nymphs and adults, which have eight legs, are darker. Larvae and nymphs are extremely small, the size of a poppy seed or smaller, and can be mistaken for a speck of dirt. Adult ticks are about the size of a sesame seed or larger.

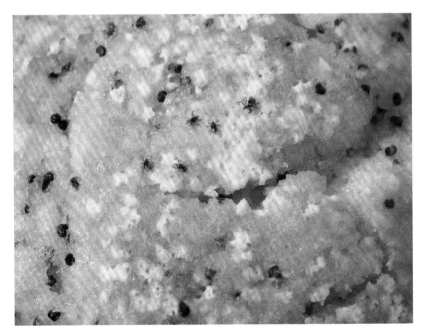

This photo demonstrates just how small larval and nymphal ticks can be — about the size of a poppy seed.

How Ticks Feed

When a tick is looking for a blood meal, it will increase its chances of finding a host by altering its behavior. Whereas a larval tick waits for a host on the ground, a hungry nymph or adult crawls to the top of a stalk of grass or shrub and exhibits "questing" behavior, where it sits with its front legs outstretched and waving, waiting for an appropriate host to wander by. For nymphs, the host is typically a small mammal, whereas adult ticks prefer bigger hosts, such as deer. When an animal (including a human) walks by, the questing tick grabs onto it with its outstretched front legs. Ticks *do not* jump or fall from trees.

Once on the animal, the tick often wanders around looking for the best place to feed. It feeds by piercing its mouthparts into the skin of the host and "plugging into" a capillary (a very small blood vessel). Though the anatomy of a tick's mouthparts differ between species, generally ticks have a few key structures that allow them to latch onto and feed on the host's blood so effectively: two palps, which move aside when feeding; two chelicerae, which cut through the skin; and a hypostome, which is a needle-like structure with barbs that point back toward the tick's body, making it difficult for the tick to become dislodged (such as when you try to remove it). While feeding, the tick secretes various chemicals that help secure it to the skin of its host and avoid detection while it feeds.

The tick continues to suck blood from the host for up to several days and may become engorged, swelling to many times its original size. A large nymph or adult tick can be nearly the size of a pea when fully engorged with blood. At this stage they are easy to spot, but it means that the tick has likely been feeding on you for several days and may have already injected you with Lyme bacteria.

A tick "quests" by stretching out its front legs and waving. ▶

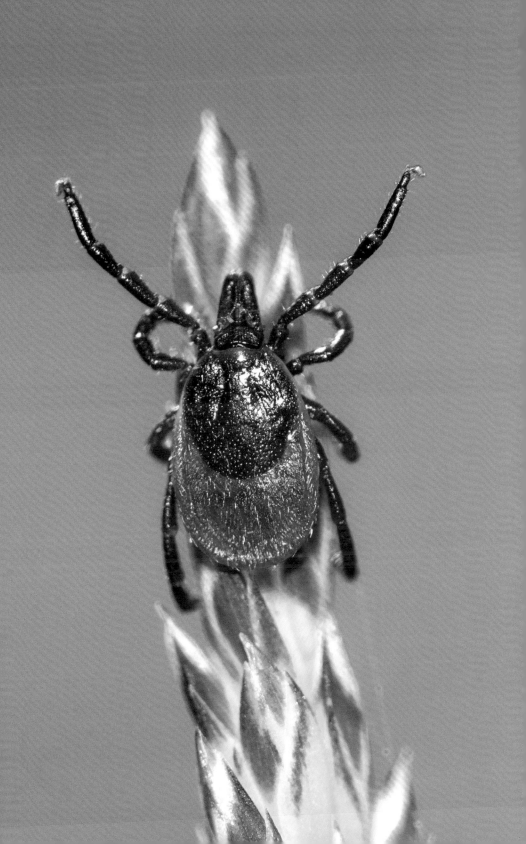

How Ticks Spread Disease

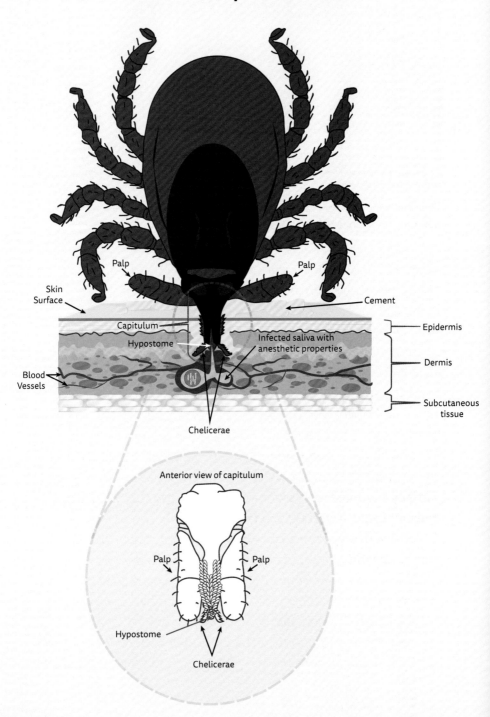

Skin Surface

Palp

Palp

Cement

Capitulum

Epidermis

Hypostome

Infected saliva with anesthetic properties

Dermis

Blood Vessels

Subcutaneous tissue

Chelicerae

Anterior view of capitulum

Palp

Palp

Hypostome

Chelicerae

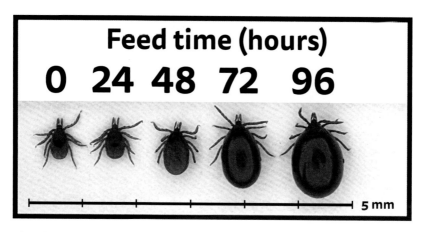

Feed time (hours)

0 24 48 72 96

5 mm

This photo shows a general scale of how large a tick can swell depending on how long it's been feeding on you.

Research has shown some interesting yet disturbing facts about the impacts *Borrelia* bacteria have on its tick host. The first is that ticks often partially engorge themselves, meaning they don't necessarily feed off their animal host until they are fully engorged. Instead, they may feed, drop off, lounge around for a bit and then look for another animal to bite and feed off. It turns out that these partially engorged ticks, which have fed repeatedly, may transmit *Borrelia* bacteria faster — possibly in under an hour — than ticks that have not fed repeatedly (Cook 2015). *So, when you are told not to worry if a tick has been feeding on you for less than 24 hours, think again.* If that tick has fed repeatedly and only partially engorged itself each time, there's a risk that the tick can transmit Lyme bacteria to you faster.

Second, ticks carrying Lyme bacteria are less prone to dehydration, meaning infected ticks are more likely to survive dry conditions compared to uninfected ticks. In other words, the hot, dry conditions that typically keep tick numbers low might not affect ticks infected with *B. burgdorferi* as much (Rawls 2017). Research also shows that ticks carrying Lyme bacteria have larger fat stores, which increases their chance of surviving harsh conditions or long spells between feeding; they are also more cold tolerant (therefore, more likely to survive the winter and be active in colder temperatures) and are able to move faster and climb higher, making them more likely to encounter an animal host, such as you (Buhner 2015).

Finally, ticks carrying *Borrelia* bacteria can eat larger blood meals, which means they may stay on their host longer. The longer a tick feeds on its host, the more likely it is to transmit the bacteria. All of these things allow the tick to be more successful at infecting multiple animal hosts, thus ensuring the proliferation of not only more ticks, but also the bacteria they transmit.

TICK HABITAT

Ticks love humidity. They don't like dry conditions, so they will seek out places where the humidity is higher. That means you are most likely to find ticks in damp places, such as in tall grass or under leaf litter on the forest floor. However, you can also encounter ticks on your front lawn even if you live in the middle of the city. The likelihood of an encounter is probably lower on an inner-city lawn than it would be if you were hiking in a forest, but just because you live in the city doesn't mean you shouldn't be doing tick checks in the spring, summer and fall after you spend time in your yard.

I live on 15 acres (6 hectares) of forested land. I have a fairly small mowed front lawn, and my backyard consists of a mix of gardens, some mowed grass, naturally shrubby/grassy areas and forest. In spring and fall, when it's damp, the ticks are really bad in my backyard, and my risk of a tick encounter is high. However, in the summer months, I barely see a tick because the soils in my area are shallow and can become very dry. Mind you, if I'm traipsing through the forest around my house in the summer, I definitely still worry about ticks. It's all about the damp spaces when it comes to ticks.

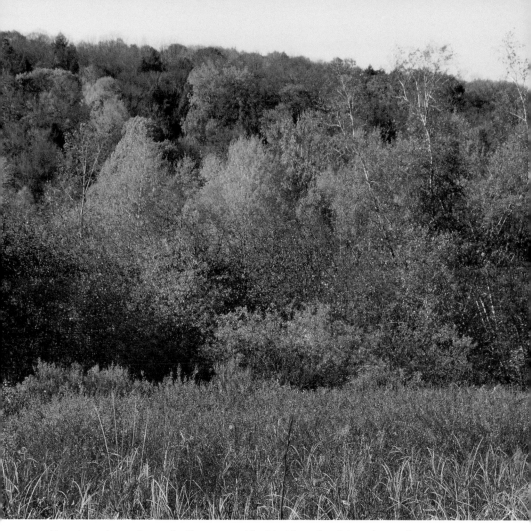

Forests and meadows of tall grass are ideal habitats for ticks, who prefer damp places.

Even if you experience dry summers like me, it doesn't mean the ticks die off. The black-legged tick is a tough little creature. Its hard exoskeleton allows it to withstand dry conditions for prolonged periods of time. It can also slow its metabolism and go into a dormant state to survive harsh conditions. Some species of ticks can even absorb water from the air by secreting a liquid from their salivary glands that absorbs moisture. Once the salivary secretion has absorbed enough water, the tick simply reingests it to get its hydration (Bowman and Sauer 2004). How's that for impressive?

Do I Need to Worry About Ticks in Winter?

The answer to this question is it depends on where you live and what your climate is like. The life cycle of the tick is highly temperature dependent, which is why climate change appears to be having such an impact on the prevalence of Lyme disease in North America. The milder and wetter our winters continue to become in eastern and central North America, the more likely it is that ticks will remain active during the winter months. There is evidence that ticks are active at temperatures as low as 36°F (2°C). So if you live in an area with mild winters, such as the Pacific coast or the southern United States, ticks will be active in winter and you need to be vigilant — using repellent and carrying out tick checks and other actions to help minimize the likelihood of a tick bite.

Over the past few years, it has not been unusual for winter temperatures to fluctuate considerably where I live in eastern Ontario — with cold spells hitting –22°F (–30°C) or lower, and within days, the temperature increasing wildly to 54°F (12°C). These warm winter days are often accompanied by rain, which melts the snow and exposes the leaf litter and vegetation, where the ticks hang out during winter. During some years my area has experienced stretches where temperatures were well above freezing for as long as a few days to a week. It is at these times when you would be most at risk of a winter encounter with a tick.

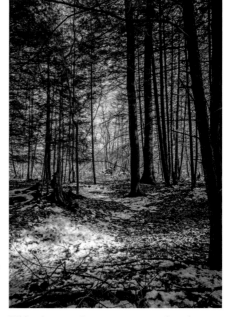

Mild and wetter winters mean you need to take precautions against ticks all year round.

Not only is it important for you to check yourself for ticks after a winter hike, but also check your pets after they have been outdoors. If you heat your house with wood in winter, you may inadvertently bring ticks into your house on firewood. Just be vigilant if you stack wood indoors. Ticks can crawl off the wood and onto you or your pets.

Given that we are most likely to encounter ticks when we are in more natural environments, such as forests and meadows, I have had people tell me that to avoid tick bites they plan to lock themselves indoors and never go hiking again. To me, this isn't a solution. Yes, ticks are a new reality that we have to deal with, but they shouldn't cause you to hide indoors. After all, the residents of Churchill, Manitoba, have learned to coexist with polar bears. If they can learn to live safely with the world's largest bears in their midst, surely we all can learn to coexist with ticks. The benefits we get from being outdoors are far too great. We just need to adopt new habits to minimize our chances of a tick bite — something we will cover in the next chapter.

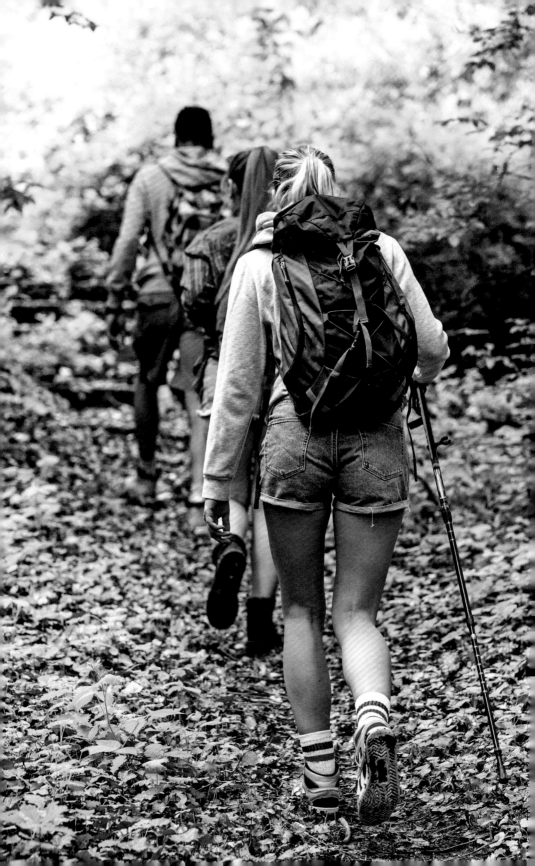

CHAPTER **3**

Reducing the Risk of a Tick Bite

There are a number of things you can do to still enjoy the outdoors and reduce your risk of a tick bite. As you'll learn in Chapter 4, if you are bitten by a tick, it isn't just Lyme disease you need to worry about. There are other tick-borne infections you can get from a tick bite, so it's important to ensure you minimize the risk of encounters with ticks and the possibility of a bite.

REPELLENTS AND INSECTICIDES

One of the best ways to prevent a tick bite is to use a repellent. The year that I found the engorged tick on my back, I did a lot of research on what repellents and insecticides were available for keeping ticks away, and I've looked into everything from repellent recipes that use essential oils to icaridin-based sprays to permethrin-infused clothing.

For all the repellents and insecticides listed, keep the containers away from children and pets, and use caution and common sense when you apply them on yourself or someone else. While

◄ The fear of ticks and tick-borne diseases shouldn't keep you from the outdoors. Simple measures can be taken to ensure you don't get bitten.

I will talk about my personal preferences, I encourage you to do your own research to make an informed decision about what repellents work best for you and your family.

Essential Oils

Essential oils have the reputation of being the more "natural" way to deter ticks, and they're definitely the most aromatically pleasant. I have made my own essential oil repellent using rose geranium (*Pelargonium graveolens*) oil and alcohol, and I have found that this repellent works well. I've read several accounts that state that rose geranium is one of the most effective essential oil repellents. I'm not sure which specific chemical in this essential oil makes it effective, but the ticks certainly don't seem to like it. I make my own spray in a 4-fluid-ounce (118-milliliter) colored glass spray bottle. (Use colored glass so that UV light from the sun doesn't break down the chemical components in the essential oil). Add about 40 drops of rose geranium oil to the bottle, and then fill half the bottle with water and the other half with alcohol (I use vodka that is 40 percent alcohol by volume; I have also heard of people using witch hazel or apple cider vinegar instead). Shake the bottle well before spraying.

You'll find other recipes on the Internet that use other essential oils or blends, such as eucalyptus, clove, citronella, cedarwood, thyme, lemongrass or peppermint. I have also seen suggestions for using oil of oregano. Interestingly, the secondary compounds in oregano are known to be antimicrobial, meaning they can kill Lyme bacteria (which is why oil of oregano is often part of the treatment for chronic Lyme disease and other tick-borne infections). However, spraying oil of oregano on your skin will likely have little or no effect on the Lyme bacteria in your bloodstream.

I suggest spraying the essential oil repellent directly onto your clothing as well as your skin. To ensure that the oil won't leave a stain on your clothing, spray a small test patch in an

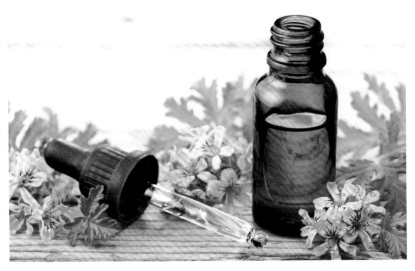

Repellents made from essential oils, such as rose geranium oil, are a fragrant alternative to store-bought repellents.

inconspicuous place first. Some people may find that essential oils can be irritating to their skin, so if you decide to apply an essential oil repellent directly to your skin, it's a good idea to dilute it in a carrier oil, such as grapeseed oil or coconut oil, and test it on a small patch of skin before using it on the rest of your body.

The main issue I find with essential oil repellents is that I have to reapply them frequently (every 1 to 2 hours) as they tend to wear off quickly, so I carry a small bottle of my homemade repellent with me when I'm outside and reapply it about once an hour.

Essential Oils and Cats

Many essential oils can be toxic to cats, so please use caution if you make your own essential oil tick repellent. Exposing a cat to essential oils can lead to serious liver damage and failure, seizures or death, regardless of whether the oils are used internally, applied to the skin or inhaled.

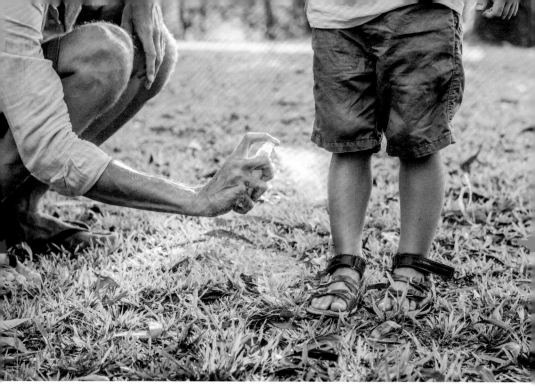

Spraying yourself with repellent from the knees down every time you go outside will ensure you're protected while doing your day-to-day activities.

Icaridin-Based Repellents

The best repellents I've tried are those that contain the active ingredient icaridin, also referred to as picaridin. My local hardware store carries it, and it can be found in most stores that carry insect repellent, or online. Icaridin repellent with a 20 percent concentration is generally effective at repelling ticks (and mosquitoes) for 12 hours, and it offers 10-hour protection from black flies.

I spray it on my legs (from the knees down) and feet every morning before I take my dog outside. This way I am protected for the day, whether I'm gardening, mowing the lawn or just walking around in the backyard. If I go for a walk in the woods, I spray it all over, including my upper body, because I may brush up against tree limbs or shrubs where ticks are waiting.

In my experience, most ticks get on me by climbing onto my shoes and then crawling up to find a place to feed, so spraying lots of repellent on my legs from the knee down seems to work well at keeping ticks off. However, it's important for you to do what you are most comfortable with. If you think you need to spray yourself all over, do it.

Icaridin is generally described as being a safe ingredient and is approved for use in repellents with up to 20 percent concentration (the concentration will determine how long the product is effective for). The Public Health Agency of Canada's Committee to Advise on Tropical Medicine and Travel recommends using icaridin-based repellents for travelers six months and older. Icaridin has fewer cautions than DEET-based repellents, is nonscented (I find it has a slight scent, but it is very tolerable, especially compared to DEET) and non-oily, and it won't dissolve plastic or synthetic materials the way DEET does.

Of course, caution and common sense should always be exercised with whatever repellent you're spraying yourself with. The Material Safety Data Sheet (MSDS) for icaridin states that the repellent is not a known carcinogen but warns that a 20 percent repellent solution (which also contains ethanol and propylene glycol) can cause eye or skin irritation. It can also cause irritation if inhaled, and ingesting it may cause a headache, nausea, vomiting and weakness as well as liver issues (probably due to the ethanol in the repellent). Chronic exposure to icaridin can cause defatting dermatitis, which results in drying, cracking and whitening of the skin.

Icaridin-based products are my preferred repellents, but it is up to you to decide what you feel comfortable using, especially if you have preexisting sensitivities to certain chemical compounds.

DEET-Based Repellents

DEET is the active ingredient in many insect repellents, including lotions and sprays. It repels ticks, mosquitoes and black flies. As the concentration of DEET increases, so does the duration of protection. So, for example, a 7 percent concentration will give you up to 90 minutes of protection, while a 30 percent concentration will give you up to 10 hours of protection.

According to the United States Environmental Protection Agency (EPA) website, formulations for DEET-based bug repellent products can contain up to a 99 percent concentration, and the agency concluded in a 2014 assessment that the normal use of DEET does not present health concerns to the general population, including children. As with all repellents, be sure to follow label directions and use common sense when applying on yourself or someone else.

According to its MSDS, DEET is listed as having the possibility of causing neurological damage if used in large quantities, although I'm not sure that most backyard gardeners, campers and hikers would use large enough quantities of DEET to cause problems. The MSDS also states that DEET at a concentration of 95 percent or higher can cause skin irritation and sensitization, eye irritation and gastrointestinal irritation (including nausea, vomiting and diarrhea), and it can be harmful if swallowed. Inhaling it may cause respiratory tract irritation or irritation of the mucous membranes. For repeated and prolonged exposure to DEET, the MSDS warns that it may cause adverse reproductive effects and may produce erythremia (an increase in the number of red blood cells), bullous eruptions, contact urticaria (localized swelling and redness of the skin), muscle cramping, slurred speech, tremors, seizures or coma.

As a photographer and field biologist, I've also found that DEET will dissolve certain plastics, such as those used for camera or binocular straps. I personally don't like DEET, and I find that its effectiveness as a repellent is shorter than that of icaridin.

Permethrin

Permethrin is an insecticide that you may have heard mentioned as a tick deterrent. It is designed to kill ticks and insects if they

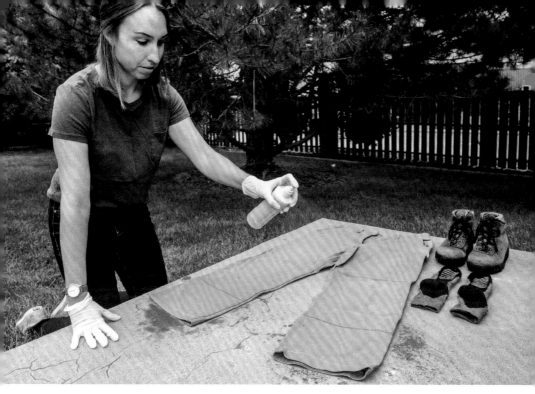

Be sure to take proper safety precautions while applying permethrin to your clothes and gear.

touch or eat it, affecting their nervous systems and causing muscle spasms, paralysis and death. It is also an active ingredient in some dog flea and tick shampoos and topical medications for scabies and lice.

Permethrin spray should never be applied directly on the skin. Instead, it should only be used to treat your clothing and gear, and you should wait for the spray to dry before touching your clothes. The EPA also recommends washing permethrin-treated clothing separately from other clothing.

The spray form currently cannot be purchased commercially in Canada, but it is widely available in the United States. In Canada (as well as in the United States) you can buy clothes, including shirts, pants and shorts, that are pretreated with permethrin, and the treatment is said to last on these items for 70 washes.

Personally, I don't use permethrin due to its potential toxicity. Its MSDS lists it as a potential mutagen (a substance that can alter

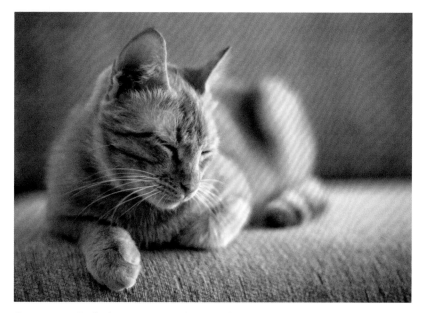

Cats are particularly sensitive to the pyrethroids in permethrin, so be careful about using permethrin and permethrin-treated clothing around your feline friends.

or damage DNA) and a tumor-causing agent. Its MSDS also states that it is harmful if swallowed or inhaled and can cause an allergic reaction on the skin or be irritating to the skin. It is also very toxic to aquatic life, so if you live rurally and are on a septic system, regularly using permethrin-treated clothing is probably not a good idea since the permethrin that washes off when you clean your clothes will end up in your septic system and eventually out in the environment, including groundwater and surface water. In addition to its potential nasty effects on humans and aquatic life, it is also highly toxic to cats, and with two cats in my household, I don't want to risk it. Finally, permethrin is toxic to bees, so do not spray your clothing with it while standing beside your flower garden.

For more information, I would highly recommend you search for the MSDS for whatever permethrin product you are considering using so that you understand the health risks.

Cats and Permethrin

Permethrin is particularly poisonous to cats because their livers are unable to metabolize (break down) the active chemicals in it, called pyrethroids. Out of caution, you should keep any permethrin products, including permethrin-treated clothes, away from cats and wash permethrin-treated clothing separately from any cat bedding or things that your cats might be exposed to. Cats can also come into contact with permethrin through dog flea and tick shampoos or topical products, either by having the product applied directly to their bodies or being exposed to a dog recently treated with a pyrethroid product. If you suspect your cat has been exposed to permethrin or another pyrethroid product, take them to a veterinarian immediately.

TICK CHECKS

Checking for ticks is one habit that I highly recommend everyone adopt, whether you live rurally or in the city. I cannot emphasize this enough. As I mentioned previously, depending on where you live, tick densities are likely to be considerably lower on a city lawn than they are in the leaf litter on a forest floor, but that doesn't mean you won't encounter a tick on your lawn.

Tick checks are easy to do and should become a part of your daily routine. I recommend performing tick checks at least twice a day: Before bed do a full-body tick check to make sure there are no ticks crawling on you or feeding, and do the same thorough check when you get up in the morning. Why twice? Because if you missed the tick in the evening and it has been feeding on you overnight, it will likely be bigger in the morning because it is more engorged with blood, which means it will be easier to spot. It is critical to remove a tick as soon as you find it.

In terms of where to look when doing a full-body tick check, the answer is… everywhere! And I do mean *everywhere*. Remember, ticks like moist places, so you can imagine some of the places they may choose to latch onto you. When a tick first crawls onto

Where to Check for Ticks

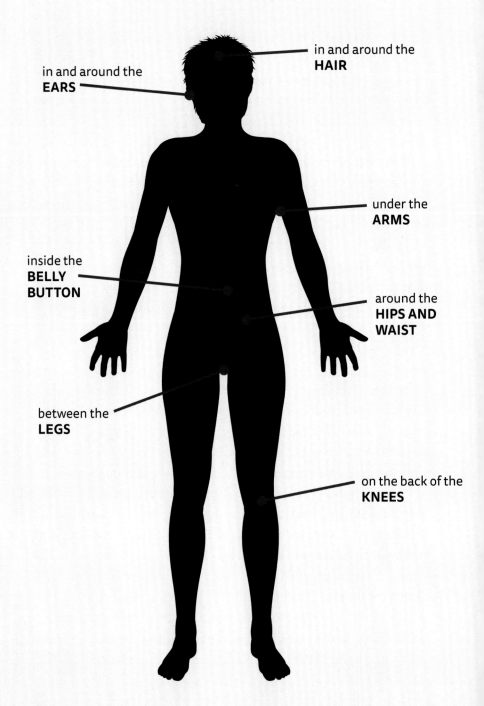

in and around the
HAIR

in and around the
EARS

under the
ARMS

inside the
BELLY BUTTON

around the
HIPS AND WAIST

between the
LEGS

on the back of the
KNEES

your body, it looks for the best place to "plug in" to begin feeding. They tend to look for places where your skin is thinner. Ticks have been known to park themselves under bra straps, underwear bands, pant waistbands and similar places, so it's important to check out these areas of your body carefully. Also be sure to look in less-obvious places, such as behind your ears, on your scalp, in your armpits, under your breasts, behind your knees, between your toes, in your belly button, and, yes, around those nether regions.

Believe it or not, I recently found a tick in the outer corner crease of my eyelid. It was small and so well hidden in the crease that nobody saw it until several hours later, when it was engorged enough to be visible.

In addition to my nighttime and morning tick checks, I also look for ticks immediately after coming inside from outdoor activities, such as hiking and gardening. It's also a good idea to examine your clothes and any gear you may have had outdoors with you.

Checking Kids

It is really important to do a thorough tick check on your kids if they have been outside. Because a nymph tick can be the size of a poppy seed, it can be easy to miss. Teens will probably want to do their own tick check, but be sure to assist younger kids so that they don't miss any places. This way, your kids will also learn where to look, and you will help them develop this important twice-daily habit. Be sure to carefully check your child's scalp. It's easy for a tick to go undetected under thick hair. You might even consider using a louse comb, which is a very fine-toothed comb, to catch any ticks that you simply can't see.

Checking Pets

Unfortunately, it's possible for your pets to unknowingly bring ticks into the house, and then when you curl up on the couch with your cat or dog, the tick can migrate from your pet onto you. This

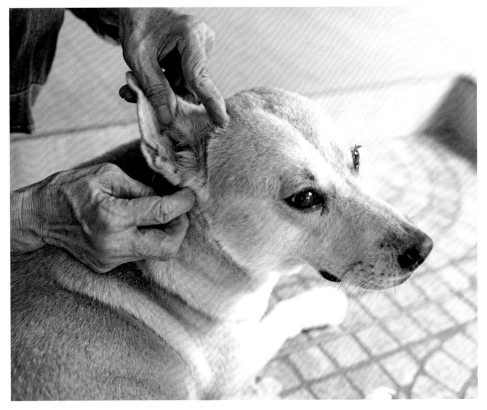

A thorough tick check after your pet has been outside is important for both your animal and you.

is why it is increasingly necessary to treat pets with preventative treatments nearly all year long — especially since, as we covered in the previous chapter, some ticks can bite even in the winter.

In addition to giving your pet vet-recommended preventative treatments, you should also do tick checks on them every time they come inside from being outdoors. In general, ticks look for areas where the skin is thinner, so they often migrate to an animal's face. I most often find ticks on the top of my dog's head or around her eyes. I have also found ticks on her belly. To check your pet, run your fingers through your pet's fur and feel for any slight bumps. Then check in and around the ears, around the

Where to Check for Ticks on Your Pet

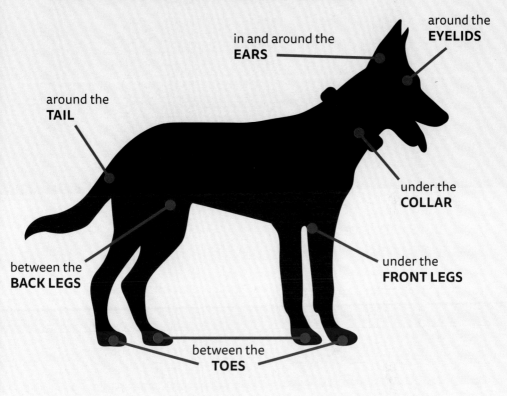

in and around the
EARS

around the
EYELIDS

around the
TAIL

under the
COLLAR

between the
BACK LEGS

under the
FRONT LEGS

between the
TOES

eyelids, under the collar, under the front legs, between the back legs, between the toes and around the tail.

If you find a tick, remove it as soon as possible.

If your pet shares your bed, it's a good idea to ensure you perform a tick check on yourself in the morning, even if your pet primarily lives indoors. Both of my cats are indoor cats, but they do spend time on my screened porch. I have discovered that at night, mice can find their way onto the porch, and with small rodents also come ticks. If a tick drops off a mouse that was on the porch, and the tick finds its way onto one of my cats, then the cat can easily bring the tick indoors and into my bed. I'm certain this is how I got my tick bite in spring 2019. My point here is that your pets can bring ticks inside, and if you sleep with your pets or spend a lot of time in close contact with them, it is possible for you to "inherit" ticks from them.

The way I look at it, the few minutes it takes to do a tick check on both you and your pet are worth it in the long term. The pain and suffering associated with Lyme disease and other tick-borne diseases make this twice-daily habit so important.

SHOWERS AND BATHS

When I'm outside in places where I could encounter a tick, the first thing I do when I come inside is have a shower or a soak in the hot tub. Despite loving humidity, ticks don't like water. If there is a tick on you that is not feeding (meaning, its mouthparts are not embedded in your skin), then it will hop off you as soon as water hits it. I have been in the shower, not knowing a tick was on me, felt a prick, looked down and watched a tick go down the drain. Given that larval and nymphal ticks can be tiny and look like specks of dirt, having a quick shower or soak is, in my experience, one of the best ways to ensure you get any crawling ticks off your body. Before I hop in the shower or tub, I still do a full-body tick check.

If you don't want to have a shower or bath and you have a pool or hot tub, have a quick swim or soak. Or if you're at a cottage on a lake, you can dunk yourself under the water for a few minutes.

Bathing only helps to remove ticks that haven't started feeding. When I found the fully engorged tick on my back, I tried soaking it off in the hot tub. That didn't work. In retrospect, I think it was a bad idea because if the tick had eventually drowned, the process may have caused it to regurgitate, meaning it could have potentially transmitted even more *Borrelia* bacteria or other microbes. Trying to soak the tick off was more of an act of panic and desperation rather than rational thinking on my part.

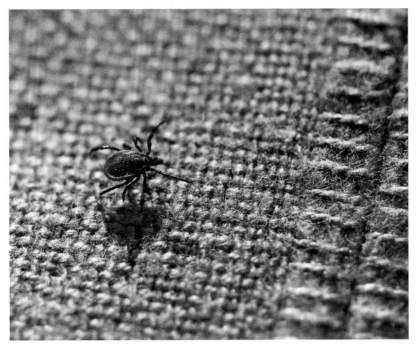

Ticks you've picked up outside may still be lurking on your clothes, so it's recommended you remove your clothes right when you get in and throw them in the washer or dryer.

CLOTHES IN THE DRYER

While I'm in the shower or having a soak, I also put the clothes I was just wearing in the dryer on high heat for 20 minutes. This is likely to kill any ticks that might be hiding in my clothing. If you simply put your dirty clothes in the laundry hamper, any ticks on your clothes may simply escape the hamper and crawl around your house looking for a host. You can also wash your clothes immediately, but if you don't want to do that, at least put your clothes in the dryer. I don't know if the heat from the dryer is enough to kill 100 percent of hardy adult ticks that may be lurking in your clothes, but it should certainly kill larvae and nymphs, which are smaller and harder to see.

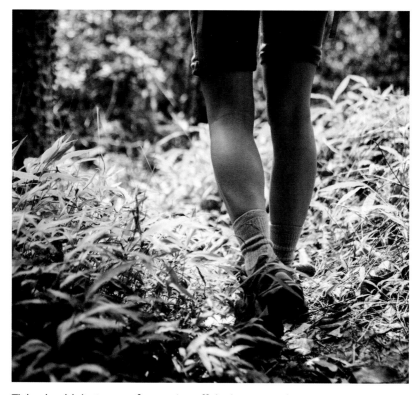

Ticks shouldn't stop you from going off the beaten path.

OTHER METHODS

What else can you do to minimize the chances of being bitten by a tick? I certainly think using common sense and vigilance are two of your best tools when dealing with tick prevention.

For example, public health units generally recommend people stick to trails when out hiking. Although this may reduce the chances of tick bite, in my view it may also reduce your enjoyment of nature. It's up to you to decide what you are comfortable with. When I'm hiking, I go off trail, but I also ensure I have applied icaridin spray before hiking and do tick checks, have a shower and put my clothes in the dryer immediately after my hike. In other words, by being vigilant about applying repellents and checking for ticks after every time I go outside, I am minimizing my risk of being bitten.

Yard Maintenance

If you're trying to limit tick populations in your yard, fairly simple yard maintenance can help. The Connecticut Agricultural Experiment Station developed the *Tick Management Handbook*, and here are some of their suggestions for yards:

- Rake and remove dead leaves from the lawn immediately surrounding your house, particularly in early spring. Because ticks like moist environments, they love to hang out in leaf litter.
- Mow the lawn immediately surrounding your house regularly and clear tall grasses and brush around the yard.
- If you live on the edge of woodlands, keep high-use features, such as lawns and playgrounds, at least 3 yards (2.7 meters) from the forest edge.
- Trim back tree branches and shrubs to allow more sunlight into your yard. Bright, sunny areas are hotter and drier and less likely to harbor ticks.

I want to emphasize that your goal should not be to turn your yard into a sterile environment that lacks biodiversity. Be mindful that by raking up leaves, you are removing critical overwintering habitat for many species of native insects — insects that will be food for baby birds in spring. So please, do not rake up every leaf on your property, and do not cut down your trees. Doing so will have more of a devastating effect on your yard's biodiversity than its tick population.

A far more balanced approach is to ensure that the area immediately surrounding your house, where you and your family are most likely to walk and play, consists of short grass, stone or other materials that ticks don't like. I live rurally, surrounded by forests. I don't cut down my trees; I simply keep my front and back lawns reasonably leaf-free, keep my grass reasonably short, put wood mulch on my garden beds, and, for the rest of my property, just let nature do its thing.

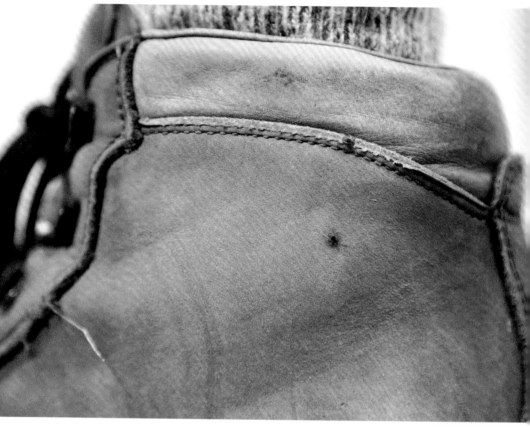

Ticks tend to be easier to spot on lighter-colored shoes and clothes.

We need to enjoy nature and learn to live in harmony with it. Like it or not, ticks are here to stay, but hiding inside your house or turning your yard into a sterile environment that supports no biodiversity is not the answer.

Clothing Choices

Public health agencies variously recommend wearing light-colored clothing, long-sleeved shirts and long pants, usually with the pant legs tucked into your socks.

I think wearing light-colored clothing is a reasonable idea, as it will help you spot any ticks that may be crawling on your clothes.

As for the other recommendations, it's really up to your personal preference and comfort level. I personally find long-sleeved shirts and long pants too hot for me, particularly during the humid summers of eastern Ontario. When I hike in the woods, I wear shorts, short socks and hiking boots or shoes, and I make sure to spray my boots and socks well with an icaridin-based repellent. Depending on whether I will be walking through shrubby areas and over forest undergrowth, I may also spray the rest of my body. I also wear shorts because, to be frank, I want to see the tick crawling on me (rather than have it crawl up my leg, hidden under my pants), so that I can pick it off. This is purely my own approach.

To me, one potential issue with long pants tucked into socks is that ticks look for tight spots to crawl into, areas where clothing is tight against your skin, which is why you often discover tick bites under bra straps, underwear bands and pant waistbands. My worry is if that if I tuck my pant legs into my socks, I might be creating a tight, cozy place for a tick to settle down for dinner. As well, I might not see those hitchhikers under my socks until I take off my clothes when I get home. Of course, this is my own personal take on this issue. I can't emphasize enough that you must decide what you feel most comfortable with and what makes sense to you and your own lifestyle.

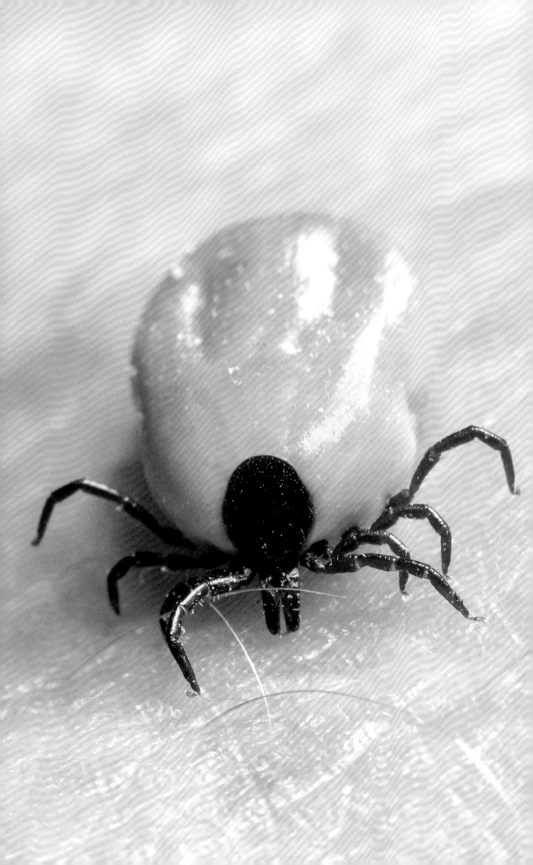

CHAPTER **4**

What If I'm Bitten?

HOW TO REMOVE A TICK

If you do find a tick on you, it is extremely important that you remove it *as soon as possible*. The longer the tick feeds on you, the greater the chance that it will transmit the Lyme bacteria (and any other microbes it is carrying) to you.

One of the most important things about tick removal is to ensure you remove the head, not just the body. *Borrelia* bacteria and other microbes reside in the tick's gut but move to the salivary glands as it feeds. The salivary glands are associated with the mouthparts on the head, so if you leave the head embedded in your skin, microbes could still be transmitted to you, at least for a little while.

Use a clean pair of fine-tipped tweezers to pull the tick out. Be sure to grasp the tick as close to the skin as possible to ensure you're gripping its head. Next, pull steadily and firmly to get it out. Remember that ticks are masters at staying attached to you because they have backward-pointing barbs on their mouthparts and secrete a cement, of sorts, to keep themselves glued onto you,

◄ An engorged tick after a blood meal.

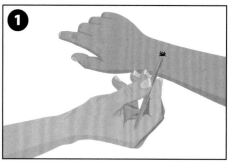
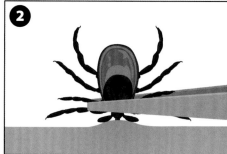
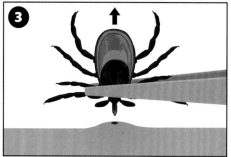
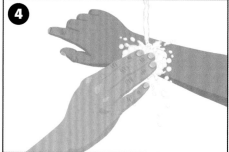

If you find a biting tick, follow these directions:

❶ Remove the tick using a clean pair of fine-tipped tweezers or a tick remover.

❷ Grasp the tick as close to the skin's surface as possible.

❸ Pull upward with steady, even pressure. Don't twist or jerk the tick as you can risk detaching it from its mouthparts.

❹ Clean the bite area and your hands thoroughly with rubbing alcohol or soap and water.

so you have to pull firmly. I have also heard that if you disturb the tick while it's feeding, the disturbance might cause it to regurgitate. So when you pull the tick out, try to do it with one good pull.

If you pull out the tick but its head and mouthparts are still embedded in your skin, try to remove them with your tweezers. If you're still unable to remove them, contact your doctor.

You can also use a tick remover to pull out the feeding tick. There are a few different types available. One of the most popular tools that works well is shaped like a hockey stick and has a head on it with a slot. You slide the tick into the slot and pull hard. This

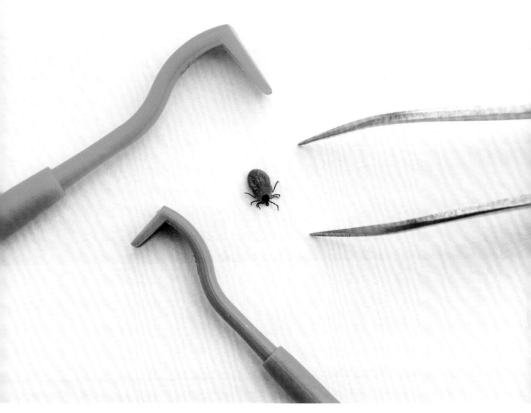

There are a variety of tick removers on the market. The key is finding a tool that can grasp the tick as closely to the skin surface as possible.

kind of tick remover ensures that the tick is being grasped close to the skin, so it is more likely that the entire head will be removed.

You can use tick removers to take ticks off your pets as well. Your local veterinary clinic will likely sell them. It is good to have a few on hand: one for at home and one that goes with you on hikes or walks in case you find a tick on you or your pet while you're out.

Another very important caution is that you should not apply any substance to the tick to kill it while it is still attached and feeding on you. I have heard of people smearing petroleum jelly over the tick, or painting it with clear nail polish. This is a really bad idea. Yes, you will kill the tick, but applying a substance may make the tick regurgitate as it dies, increasing the likelihood of it transmitting *Borrelia* or other microbes to you. Your best course of action is to simply remove the tick with tweezers or a tick remover.

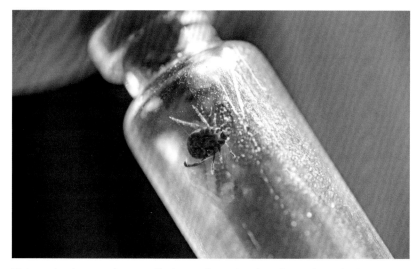

Tick testing is a good way to find out what microbes that tick might have transferred to you or your pet, so be sure to keep the tick.

Once you have removed the tick, I highly recommend that you put it in a glass vial in the fridge and then send it off for testing. When I had a tick removed from my back at my local hospital, I brought a vial with me so I could keep the tick and get it tested.

Where to Get Your Ticks Tested

In Canada:
Geneticks (geneticks.ca)

In the United States:
Fry Laboratories (frylabs.com)
TickCheck (tickcheck.com)
Ticknology (ticknology.org)

The Lyme Disease Association in the United States has a great resource page that lists places in the U.S. where you can get your tick tested, including a listing by state. Use your smartphone camera to scan the QR code above or visit lymediseaseassociation.org /about-lyme/tick-removal-a-testing/tick-testing-2/

The hospital told me there was nowhere to get it tested, but this is simply not true. Federal testing labs can test for the presence of microbes, but it is unlikely that your doctor will submit your tick for testing. Instead, you can send it yourself to a private lab, and the testing is usually done for a reasonable fee (see the box on page 76).

How Infection Occurs

When a tick bites you it pierces your skin with its sucking mouth-parts. It plugs into one of your capillaries and lets blood freely flow into its gut. During this process the tick secretes a wonderful cocktail of chemicals into you, its host (Francischetti et al. 2009).

All of these chemicals play some role in allowing the tick to feed for up to several days. One of these chemicals prevents your blood from clotting, so the blood continues to flow into the tick for the duration of its feeding. There is also a chemical that acts as an anesthetic so that you don't feel the tick biting. If you felt the tick biting, much like when you feel a mosquito biting, you would immediately be alerted to the bite and remove the tick. However, the anesthetic lets the tick stealthily feed at your expense and without your knowledge for days.

There might be rare circumstances when you do feel the tick biting. This happened to me when I was bitten in the crease of my eyelid. I didn't feel the tick biting me initially, but after it had been feeding for several hours I began to feel some pain on my eyelid. When the pain became intense, I looked in the mirror and discovered the tick. Once it was removed, I experienced extreme pain at the bite site as well as considerable swelling. Over the next few days the pain turned into a burning sensation, and a few days later the sensations and swelling subsided.

Tick saliva also contains chemicals that suppress your immune system so that your body doesn't react to the foreign objects (i.e., the tick's mouthparts) jabbed into your skin or the other chemicals in its saliva. The tick also secretes a chemical that acts like a glue to keep its mouthparts embedded in your skin so that it can continue to feed. The sharp barbs on its mouthparts also ensure that it stays plugged into its host until it decides to drop off.

Bacteria generally hang out in the gut of an infected tick. When the tick starts feeding, the Lyme bacteria move from the tick's midgut into its salivary glands and are then transmitted into the host during the tick's blood meal. When the bacteria are first transmitted, they are concentrated under the skin at the site of the bite. Over the next two to four weeks, the bacteria disseminate from the bite site into the bloodstream and then to other parts of the body, particularly the central nervous system, gastrointestinal system, heart and joints. (Children often exhibit gastrointestinal problems as one of their main symptoms of Lyme disease.) If the human host is not treated by antibiotics, the bacteria reproduce and the infection grows. As the bacteria multiply, they manipulate the immune system, causing inflammation and consequently, the symptoms of Lyme disease. The spirochetal (corkscrew-shaped) form of the bacterium, which is present in the bloodstream for a relatively short time following the tick bite, can also burrow into tissues. By burrowing into tissues, such as the collagen in your joints, the bacteria can avoid the effects of antibiotics while feeding on the nutrients released when your tissues are broken down by your immune system's inflammatory response to the bacteria. This is one of the ways that Lyme bacteria hijack your immune system and use it to their advantage. Lyme bacteria have the ability to change shape. When they encounter unfavorable conditions in their environment, such as antibiotics or changes in pH, they can change from the spirochetal form to a "persister" form, such as a round-body form, which has a lower metabolic rate and can go on in a dormant state for months or even years.

Not everyone bitten by a tick becomes ill. If you have a healthy immune system that kills off the infection, then your immune system has done its job in protecting you. However, certain conditions such as stress, aging, hormonal changes and other factors can affect your immune system and cause it to not function as well as it should. If this happens, your body may not be able to completely kill off the Lyme bacteria but is instead able to keep the infection at a low level, where it may cause little or no illness until months or even years later, when your immune system is no longer able to keep the infection at bay. One of the challenges with this scenario is that Lyme disease is often not suspected as the cause of illness because the tick bite was so long ago and probably long forgotten (if it was noticed at all). This is why piecing together the history of a patient is such an important part of a diagnosis. As I'll explain later, diagnosing Lyme disease sometimes requires detective work.

Keep a Symptom Diary

One of the best pieces of advice I was given was to keep a diary of my symptoms. When I was bitten in spring 2019, I recorded the date the tick was removed and kept a diary of my symptoms for several months. I became ill three days after that tick was removed from my back, and my symptom diary became an important piece of the puzzle that my family doctor used to make a clinical diagnosis of Lyme disease.

If you are bitten by a tick or suspect that you have Lyme disease, I highly recommend that you create your own diary in which you list the date of your tick bite (if you saw the tick, or at least estimate the potential date if you didn't see it), and each day record any symptoms you notice. Do this daily. Symptoms can come and go and change in intensity over time. It would also be a good idea to take pictures of any bites or rashes you find, especially if you cannot see a doctor right away. Be sure to take your symptom diary and any photos to your appointment with your doctor. Your doctor will need this information, and it will likely play a critical role in receiving a diagnosis.

STAGES AND SYMPTOMS OF LYME DISEASE

It is critical to know the stages and symptoms of Lyme disease and, if you suspect you might have Lyme, to track your symptoms over time. The symptoms one person experiences may be different from those of someone else, and symptoms also vary with different stages of the disease and even with the species or strain of *Borrelia* with which you were infected (Sertour et al. 2018). The presence of coinfections such as *Bartonella* and/or *Babesia* can affect the suite of symptoms experienced. Symptoms can also appear quickly or slowly and wax and wane over time, so it's important to monitor how you're feeling each day.

Lyme disease has been described as the great imitator because the symptoms in both the early and late stages of the disease are shared by a whole suite of other chronic diseases and conditions. This is one key reason why Lyme disease can be challenging to diagnose and why a patient's history and risk of exposure to ticks and Lyme disease play such an important role in diagnosis.

There are three key stages of Lyme disease, and the following are the most common symptoms during each stage. Knowing what stage of disease you are in can help determine the most appropriate course of treatment.

Early Localized Lyme Disease
(up to four weeks after a tick bite)

During this stage the bacteria move from the skin at the site of the bite to other parts of the body. This stage is the critical time to treat Lyme disease to give a patient the best chance of eradicating the infection. However, it can be difficult to diagnose Lyme this early as symptoms may or may not be noticeable at this time and antibodies may not have yet formed, which would result in a negative serologic test.

- **Flu-like symptoms:** Early-stage Lyme disease usually presents with symptoms very similar to that of the flu. This includes fever, chills, headache, fatigue, muscle and joint aches and swollen lymph nodes. Experiencing flu-like symptoms in summer, outside the typical flu season, should be seen as a red flag for the possibility of Lyme disease. This has been somewhat complicated with the emergence of COVID-19. Some symptoms of COVID-19 overlap with those of early-localized Lyme, so you may need to be tested for COVID-19 immediately to rule it out.

- **A rash, such as *erythema migrans*:** *Erythema migrans* (EM), also known as the bull's-eye rash, is a solid red, circular rash with an outer ring that can appear first at the bite site. However, I must emphasize that the bull's-eye rash is seen in as few as 9 percent of Lyme cases (Stonehouse et al. 2010). More commonly (in over 50 percent of cases) a solid red area on the skin is seen instead (Stonehouse et al. 2010). The solid red patch can be flat or slightly raised (see the photos on page 82 for examples of different Lyme rashes). Note that many people (such as me) have been bitten by a tick and developed no rash at all, or the rash was present for a short period of time and wasn't noticed.

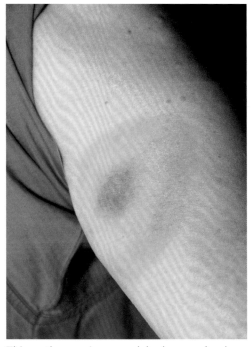

This *erythema migrans* rash looks very clearly like a bull's eye; however, studies have shown that this specific type of rash occurs in as few as 9 percent of cases.

Examples of Lyme Disease Rashes

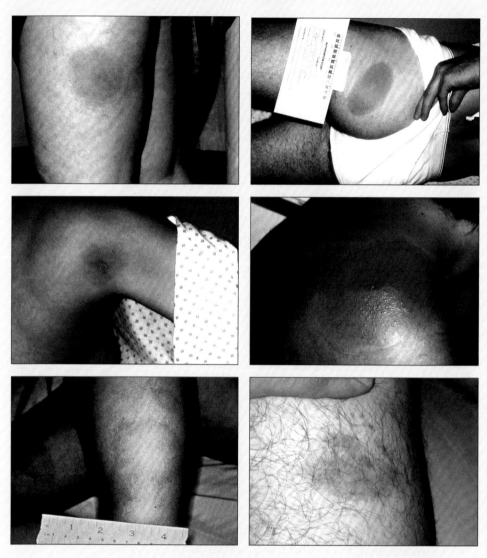

As you can see from the above photos, rashes from a *Borrelia*-infected tick have a wide variety of forms. They include disseminated lesions, blistering lesions, uniformly red lesions, blue-red lesions, oval lesions and oddly-shaped lesions, among others. You can see more examples of Lyme disease rashes by scanning the QR code or visiting cdc.gov/lyme/signs_symptoms /rashes.html

Early Disseminated Lyme Disease (one to four months after a tick bite)

During this stage the bacteria move through the bloodstream and end up in various organs and tissues around the body, especially the central nervous system, heart, joints and the gut. When the Lyme bacteria primarily attack the central nervous system, they cause neurological and psychiatric symptoms called neuroborreliosis. When they primarily attack the heart, the result is Lyme carditis, a dangerous condition in which the heart's rhythm is disrupted. When the bacteria primarily attack the joints, the result is Lyme arthritis. Children often exhibit gastrointestinal problems as one of the symptoms of Lyme. Symptoms at this stage *may* include the following:

- Headaches
- Neck stiffness
- **Arthritis with severe joint pain and possible swelling:** This usually occurs in the knees and other large joints. The joint pain typically migrates, which means that the location of the pain can vary from day to day.
- Intermittent pain in tendons, muscles and bones
- Shooting pain, numbness or tingling in the hands or feet
- Night sweats or chills
- Episodes of dizziness or shortness of breath
- Nausea
- Sore throat and/or swollen lymph nodes
- **Bell's palsy:** This is a form of partial paralysis of the facial muscles on one side of the face.
- **Heart palpitations or irregular heartbeat:** These may be symptoms of Lyme carditis, which can be life-threatening. (See pages 89–90 to learn more about Lyme carditis.)
- **Rash:** *Erythema migrans* or a solid red, circular rash may appear at the bite site or on other areas of the body. Once again, remember that a rash may be completely absent or not appear as a bull's eye. Rashes may occur on the body other than where the bite occurred, especially several days after the bite.

Late Disseminated Lyme Disease/Chronic Lyme Disease (four months to years after a tick bite)

If Lyme disease goes untreated, by the time the infection has reached the late disseminated stage, it is known as chronic, or persister, Lyme disease. Chronic Lyme disease is a multisystem infectious disease, meaning that it affects several organ systems simultaneously. As a result, the list of symptoms of late-stage Lyme disease may be long and may overlap with those of many other diseases. Lyme has been misdiagnosed as chronic fatigue syndrome, multiple sclerosis (MS), lupus, fibromyalgia, rheumatoid arthritis, amyotrophic lateral sclerosis (ALS, or Lou Gehrig's disease), Parkinson's disease and Alzheimer's disease.

Chronic Lyme Versus Post-Treatment Lyme Disease Syndrome

The Infectious Diseases Society of America (IDSA) does not recognize chronic Lyme disease and instead labels the lasting symptoms as "post-treatment Lyme disease syndrome" or "post-antibiotic Lyme arthritis." The 2020 IDSA guidelines describe "post-antibiotic Lyme disease" as the lingering symptoms of Lyme disease that remain after antibiotic treatment (Lantos et al. 2021). However, contrary to the IDSA's views, the lingering symptoms are not solely a continued response by the immune system after the bacteria have been eradicated. Rather, they are the result of inadequately treated Lyme disease, in which a short course of antibiotics may have reduced the infection load but has not killed off the infection (Cameron et al. 2014). Following inadequate antibiotic treatment, after the antibiotics have been metabolized by the body, the bacteria are then free to reproduce, building the infection load back up. As a result the patient experiences more symptoms, which are often worse than the symptoms they experienced before treatment. Persistent symptoms of Lyme disease may also be due to the continued presence of round-body, or persister, forms of the Lyme bacteria, which can remain dormant for months or years, only to revert to the spirochetal form and cause an active infection.

Suspecting Lyme

If you have received a diagnosis of chronic fatigue syndrome, MS, lupus, fibromyalgia, rheumatoid arthritis, ALS, Parkinson's disease or Alzheimer's disease, and you know or suspect you were bitten by a tick or you live in a high-risk area for Lyme, consider investigating Lyme and OTBDs to eliminate them as possible causes of your symptoms.

Similar symptoms to the early disseminated Lyme disease stage may be experienced, and as the disease progresses, the following additional symptoms may also appear:

- Phantom smells
- Unexplained weight gain or loss
- Extreme fatigue
- Swollen glands or lymph nodes
- Unexplained fevers (high- or low-grade)
- Continual infections (sinus, kidney, eye, etc.)
- Migrating pain: This type of pain moves to different body parts each day.
- A general feeling of being unwell
- Low body temperature
- Sudden allergies, chemical sensitivities or food sensitivities, such as gluten or dairy intolerance
- Sensitivity to alcohol

Long-Term Impacts of Chronic Lyme Disease

Although the symptoms of Lyme disease are broad and overlap with many other diseases and medical conditions, Lyme disease often manifests in very specific ways as the disease progresses.

The body's response to the presence of Lyme bacteria results in inflammation. Specifically, the *Borrelia* bacteria manipulate cytokines (small proteins that act as immune system messengers) to generate inflammation. Cytokines are an important part of the normal immune response to infection or injury. However, the presence of too many cytokines at persistently high levels causes problems. The inflammation generated by too many cytokines can break down tissues in the joints, brain and other parts of the nervous system, as well as other organ systems (Rawls 2017). Your body's response to the *Borrelia* bacteria can also cause a cascade of other problems. When your immune system malfunctions due to the presence of the Lyme bacteria and other tick-borne diseases (OTBDs), this opens the door for infections from herpes viruses, such as Epstein-Barr, and overgrowth of gut yeast, such as *Candida*. The presence of these infections puts further strain on the immune system and disrupts proper immune function, allowing the Lyme bacteria to gain an even stronger foothold.

An important point I want to make here, and which I will discuss in more depth later, is that the multisystem infectious diseases you might experience with chronic Lyme are not always caused solely by Lyme bacteria. Multiple coinfections by other tick-borne microbes and mold toxins can contribute to the symptoms you experience. When you are bitten by a tick, there is a high likelihood that the tick is transmitting other microbes. It is critical to understand this because the presence of OTBDs can make Lyme disease much more difficult to diagnose and treat effectively and vice versa.

Below is a basic summary of the ways chronic Lyme disease (as well as OTBDs and mold toxicity) can affect your body. This is by no means a complete or exhaustive list. It is simply meant to give you an idea of the multisystem impacts of Lyme disease and other coinfections. With each of these, keep in mind that immune dysfunction and systemic inflammation caused by the Lyme bacteria and coinfections are the underlying issues affecting the various organ systems.

Lyme arthritis – Joint pain and swelling tends to be one of the most common and persistent manifestations of chronic Lyme disease,

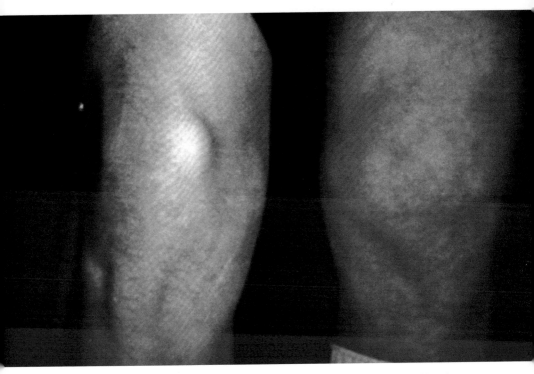

A Lyme patient with symptoms of Lyme arthritis shows significant swelling in his right knee.

and this was definitely the main symptom for me. Lyme arthritis is characterized by intermittent or persistent bouts of swelling and joint pain, with the pain moving to different joints from one day to another. Lyme arthritis can be debilitating and can be accompanied by muscle, tendon, ligament and bone pain.

Neuroborreliosis – Symptoms of Lyme disease may be concentrated in the brain and nervous system. Neuroborreliosis describes the neurological and psychiatric effects of late-stage and chronic Lyme disease. It can involve the central nervous system (which includes the brain and spinal cord) and the peripheral nervous system (which includes motor and sensory nerves, such as those in the hands and feet).

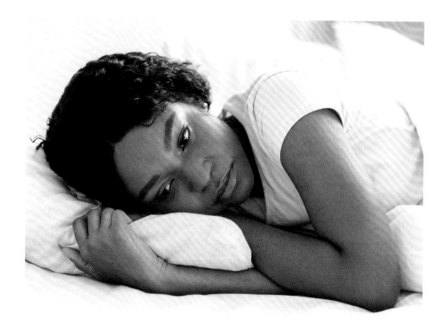

Depression, anxiety and other psychiatric and cognitive issues are key symptoms of neuroborreliosis.

As the *Borrelia* bacteria spread throughout the body, they can cross the blood-brain barrier and invade the brain, leading to inflammation of brain tissues. This inflammation can cause psychiatric issues, such as depression, anxiety or panic attacks, schizophrenia, obsessive-compulsive behaviors, mood swings, irritability and rage, as well as cognitive deficits, such as problems with short-term memory, slowed thought processing, reading and word-finding difficulties, confusion and problems concentrating. Neuroborreliosis can also manifest itself as a form of meningitis, which is an inflammation of the tissues around the brain and spinal cord, and this can be life-threatening.

Symptoms related to the peripheral nervous system include headaches; numbness; sensations of tingling, crawling, itching, burning or pricking; shooting pains; and a feeling of mild electric shocks all over the body. For some, these symptoms may come and go or be worse at night.

Muscle weakness and pain, dizziness, sensitivity to light and sound, ringing in the ears, blurred vision, changes to smell and taste and, in extreme cases, tremors and seizures can also occur. Bell's palsy, a form of partial paralysis of facial muscles on one side of the face, can be an indicator of neurological Lyme disease, and some cases of encephalitis have been linked to *Borrelia* bacteria. Lyme can also impair motor function in the limbs, leading to loss of mobility or a visible vibration or jerking of the limbs.

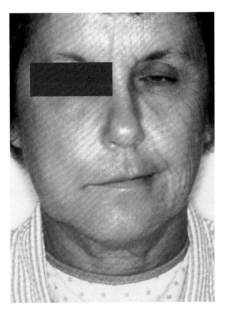

This patient who was diagnosed with Lyme disease exhibits Bell's palsy on the right side of her face.

Borrelia infections have also been linked to cases of neurodegenerative diseases, such as MS, Parkinson's, Alzheimer's and ALS, as possible causes (Rawls 2017; Horowitz 2013; Fritzsche 2005). I would urge those facing diagnosis of a neurodegenerative disease to investigate the possibility of Lyme disease because of the overlap in symptoms caused by inflammation of the brain.

Lyme carditis – Lyme carditis is much less common than the other effects of Lyme disease discussed above, affecting up to 10 percent of those with Lyme disease (Scheffold et al. 2015), but it is very serious. With Lyme carditis, the bacteria enter the tissues of the heart and affect the transmission of electrical signals between the upper and lower heart chambers (the electrical signals coordinate the beating of the heart). The resulting impaired heart function is

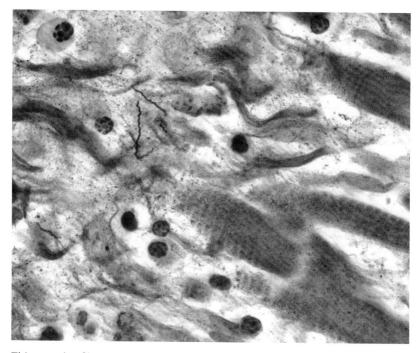

This sample of heart tissue, magnified 158 times, shows the presence of *B. burgdorferi* spirochetes.

called heart block and can be fatal if left untreated. The bacteria can also cause damage to the heart valves. Symptoms of Lyme carditis include light-headedness, fainting, shortness of breath, heart palpitations and chest pain. These may be accompanied by other Lyme disease symptoms. Lyme carditis can result in the need for a pacemaker or heart transplant. A screening tool for Lyme carditis was created by Dr. Adrian Baranchuck of Queen's University in Kingston, Ontario. His tool, called Suspicious Index in Lyme Carditis, was designed to help determine whether a patient's heart block is due to Lyme disease (Yeung and Baranchuk 2018).

Leaky gut syndrome – Disrupted immune function and the inflammation caused by Lyme bacteria (and coinfections) may lead to gastrointestinal problems, such as leaky gut syndrome.

Leaky gut occurs when the tight junctions between the cells that line the intestines weaken and pull apart, creating spaces in the lining of the intestines. These "leaks" allow bacteria, undigested food, feces and toxins to enter the bloodstream. In doing so, this situation creates more inflammation (through the release of more cytokines), which feeds the cycle of inflammation in the body, leading to chronic inflammation, and makes the person feel even sicker. Symptoms of leaky gut include bloating, gas and abdominal pain.

Another sign of leaky gut syndrome is the appearance of food sensitivities. Over the past few years, I developed sensitivities to foods that I had eaten my entire life without a problem. Gluten, cow's milk and egg whites were the biggest culprits for me, although there were other foods that I was suddenly sensitive to. I had no idea why I had developed these food sensitivities. It wasn't until I was diagnosed with chronic Lyme (and OTBDs and mold infections) that I came to understand that I had likely contracted Lyme disease years or even decades earlier and that my food sensitivities and gastrointestinal issues were the result of years of infection.

Hormone deficiencies and imbalances – Hormone deficiencies and imbalances can occur as a result of the inflammation caused by *Borrelia* bacteria and OTBDs. Lyme can affect the function of the adrenal glands, which produce stress hormones, as well as the thyroid gland and can lead to hypothyroidism (low thyroid hormone levels). The autoimmune dysfunction caused by Lyme disease can also lead to Hashimoto's thyroiditis, an autoimmune condition in which the body's own immune system attacks and destroys the thyroid gland. Abnormalities with insulin production can lead to insulin resistance, hypoglycemia and metabolic syndrome. Issues with the production of sex hormones such as estrogen and testosterone can also result from the inflammation caused by Lyme. These are just some of the hormone issues that are associated with Lyme disease and may lead to a variety of symptoms, including fatigue.

Mitochondrial dysfunction – Mitochondria are structures called organelles, and they exist in nearly every cell of the human body. You can think of mitochondria as the power stations within your cells because their role is to produce energy and power your metabolism. Mitochondrial dysfunction caused by Lyme disease is why fatigue is such a common symptom and why Lyme disease is often misdiagnosed as chronic fatigue syndrome and fibromyalgia. Correcting mitochondrial dysfunction is key to regaining energy, boosting the immune system and feeling well again.

Liver problems – The effects of Lyme disease can cause inflammation of the liver, resulting in abnormal liver chemistry. Typically, Lyme disease causes your liver to release the enzymes alanine aminotransferase (ALT), aspartate aminotransferase (AST) and gamma-glutamyl transferase (GGT) into your bloodstream. Measuring the levels of these enzymes through a blood test helps your doctor monitor your liver function. When Lyme affects the liver, it can result in symptoms such as fatigue, weight loss, nausea, muscle and joint pain and even jaundice and ascites (abnormal buildup of fluid in the abdomen), resulting from the liver's inability to get rid of toxins. These are all symptoms that can be mistaken for hepatitis, cirrhosis and other liver diseases.

Mast cell activation syndrome and other sensitivities – The immune dysfunction and inflammation caused by Lyme bacteria may also cause mast cell activation syndrome (Talkington and Nickell 1999). Mast cells are a type of immune cell that is found throughout the body. They are typically activated during allergic reactions and release histamines, but other triggers such as Lyme bacteria, other bacterial infections, mold infections, viruses, certain proteins and hormones released by the adrenal glands during times of stress can all contribute to mast cell activation syndrome (Talkington and Nickell 1999). Symptoms of mast cell activation may include typical allergy symptoms, such as itchy and watering eyes, runny nose, sneezing, itchy skin, and itchy throat. More severe cases may experience swelling of the lips, tongue and throat, wheezing and trouble breathing, low blood pressure, rapid heart rate, headache, dizziness, fatigue, and intestinal effects such as cramping, diarrhea, nausea and abdominal pain.

People with Lyme disease often develop other sensitivities as well. For example, I spontaneously developed an adverse reaction to the flu vaccine, despite having received the vaccine for over 20 years without any issues.

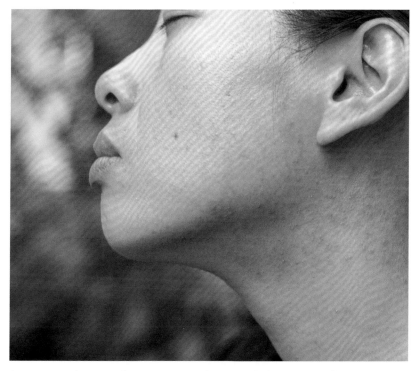

Symptoms of mast cell activation syndrome include hives and flushing skin.

Autoimmune diseases – People with chronic Lyme disease often develop autoimmune issues, in which the immune system responds inappropriately and attacks its own body. This autoimmune dysfunction triggered by Lyme bacteria and OTBDs can lead to diseases such as ulcerative colitis, Crohn's disease, MS, rheumatoid arthritis, fibromyalgia, and Hashimoto's thyroiditis (Fritzsche 2005; Chmielewska-Badora et al. 2000). The autoimmune dysfunction associated with Lyme disease has been linked to some cases of ALS, Parkinson's disease and Alzheimer's disease, as well as cancer (Pische et al. 2017; Cassarino et al. 2003; Schöllkopf et al. 2008).

As for me, I have been diagnosed with four autoimmune diseases throughout my life, and my first diagnosis was when I was just 26 years old. Because of this, I can't help wondering if I was initially infected with Lyme disease as a child or teen and that these autoimmune diseases were part of its manifestation.

For people with one or more autoimmune diseases, the links between Lyme disease and autoimmune dysfunction and diseases may be enough to spur some detective work to determine whether Lyme disease or another tick-borne infection could be involved. There is scientific evidence showing that antibiotic treatments given to patients showing early signs of MS were effective at reducing the likelihood of the patients developing clinically definitive MS (Fritzsche 2005). Of course, this isn't to say that every case of MS is rooted in Lyme disease or OTBDs. Rather, it is simply to question whether tick-borne infections could be involved.

The above descriptions of the impacts of Lyme disease on various organs and organ systems are only a rudimentary summary of how Lyme disease can affect us. The important take-home message is that chronic Lyme disease is a multisystem illness, rooted in inflammation, that can manifest itself in many ways, making it incredibly difficult to diagnose.

People experiencing chronic Lyme disease and OTBDs might

notice their symptoms wax and wane from day to day. It is common for chronic Lyme patients to have flare-ups of symptoms. The cause of these can be varied. Sometimes external factors in your environment, such as chemicals you may be sensitive to, mold spores and allergens can stress your immune system and cause it to function less effectively. They can exacerbate the already-significant systemic inflammation created by Lyme bacteria. Physical and emotional stress can also impact immune function and lead to more intense symptoms.

In my case, I have both chronic and acute Lyme disease (I was reinfected with Lyme bacteria from a tick bite in summer 2020) as well as persistent bartonellosis and a mold infection. I was also reinfected with *Babesia*, a malaria-like parasite, from my recent tick bite. I have noticed that my babesiosis symptoms (air hunger, profuse sweating on physical exertion, extreme night sweats) seem to get worse every three to four weeks, despite taking medication. This cycling of symptoms, which is a hallmark of Lyme and OTBDs, may be related to the life cycle of the *Babesia* parasite, or it may be related to my natural hormonal cycles. Regardless of the cause, I certainly experience good days and bad days, with flare-ups that can last several days to several weeks.

CONGENITAL AND PEDIATRIC LYME DISEASE

Whether Lyme disease can be passed from mother to fetus has a history of controversy. This book is not the place to delve into the details of that controversy, but it is important to acknowledge that a woman who has contracted Lyme disease can pass the *Borrelia* infection on to her unborn child. Sue Faber, of the organization LymeHope, has written a review of the peer-reviewed scientific literature and case reports published between 1985 and 2018. To read this review, visit lymehope.ca/news-and-updates/33-years-of -documentation-of-maternal-child-transmission-of-lyme-disease -and-congenital-lyme-borreliosis-a-review-by-sue-faber-rn-bscn

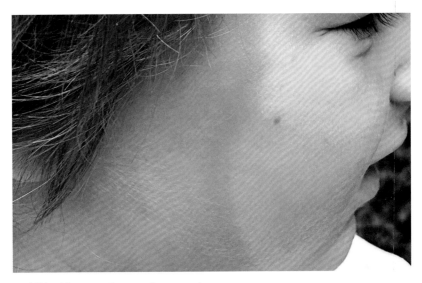

A child with an *erythema migrans* rash.

If you are pregnant or are planning on having a child and are concerned that you may have Lyme disease or a latent *Borrelia* infection from a past tick bite, I would encourage you to consult this report as well as other available resources and discuss your concerns with a Lyme-literate doctor.

Pediatric Lyme disease is a topic that has not received much attention but is no less concerning than Lyme and OTBDs in adults. If you are concerned that your child may contract Lyme disease, remember to be vigilant and do at least twice daily tick checks. On children, ticks seem to gravitate toward the scalp, so be sure to inspect your child's scalp and hair carefully — a louse comb might help catch any ticks you cannot see. Also check behind the ears, between the toes and in the bellybutton.

If you are concerned your child might already have Lyme disease, what should you look for? Diagnosing Lyme and OTBDs is a challenge at the best of times, but in children who may not be able to describe how they're feeling the way an adult can, diagnosis becomes even more difficult. Consequently, it is really important to observe your child and talk to them about how they feel.

Sexual Transmission of Lyme Disease

There is one other potential person-to-person mode of transmission of Lyme bacteria, and that is sexual transmission. A 2004 study in the *Journal of Investigative Medicine* showed the presence of *Borrelia* bacteria in vaginal secretions and semen in people who had tested positive for the presence of Lyme bacteria. The study also showed that heterosexual couples with Lyme disease were infected with the *same* strain of *Borrelia* bacteria — evidence that their infection was shared (Stricker et al. 2004).

The likelihood of sexual transmission of *Borrelia* is still being debated and needs more research; however, there is currently enough evidence to warrant caution (Stricker and Middelveen 2015; Middelveen et al. 2014). Interestingly, the Lyme bacterium is a spirochete, as is the bacterium that causes syphilis, which is sexually transmitted. Although it shouldn't be assumed that both are equally transmittable through sexual contact based simply on their shape, the evidence for *Borrelia* bacteria in semen and vaginal secretions should be enough to warrant considering protective measures to reduce the possibility of transmission.

Remember that a bull's-eye rash occurs in as few as 9 percent of cases, so don't rely on the presence of one. Do keep an eye out for other rashes, such as solid, red and oval rashes, but bear in mind no rash occurs in many cases of Lyme.

With Lyme disease, symptoms can come and go, and so this adds another level of difficulty in diagnosis. Children tend to show slightly different Lyme and OTBDs symptoms than adults. Symptoms more frequently manifest themselves as digestive issues and behavioral/neurological issues. However, children can also experience joint pain as a significant symptom. Here is a list of some of the main symptoms of Lyme and OTBDs in children:

- Fatigue
- Headaches
- Nausea, abdominal pain and diarrhea
- Joint pain

- Dizziness
- Fever/chills
- Trouble sleeping
- Noise and light sensitivity

A number of behavioral and neurological symptoms may also appear:
- Poor short-term memory
- Difficulty reading and writing
- Difficulty concentrating
- Difficulty thinking and expressing thoughts
- Confusion
- Irritability, anxiety, mood swings, outbursts and uncharacteristic behavior

Understanding the neurological and psychiatric impacts of Lyme disease in children is important because the symptoms may be misdiagnosed as an affective disorder, oppositional defiant disorder, attention deficit disorder or another cognitive issue (Tager et al. 2001). This is not to say that every one of these disorders is rooted in Lyme disease or OTBDs. However, depending on the child's history and risk of infection by tick-borne microbes, Lyme disease could be considered a possible cause.

It is not unrealistic to consider an infectious disease such as Lyme as the cause of childhood neuropsychiatric problems. Two neuropsychiatric conditions called PANDAS (pediatric autoimmune neuropsychiatric disorder associated with *Streptococcus*) and PANS (pediatric acute-onset neuropsychiatric syndrome) are both thought to result from an autoimmune reaction to infection by bacteria or viruses — *Streptococcus* in the case of PANDAS, and *Borrelia*, Epstein-Barr, H1N1 flu, *Mycoplasma* or some other infection in the case of PANS. A special issue on PANS was published in 2015 in the *Journal of Child and Adolescent Psychopharmacology* that finally gave these conditions the medical attention they deserve. What we need now is for family doctors and other health professionals to learn more about these childhood neuropsychiatric illnesses and collaborate with education professionals so that these potential illnesses are on their radar when a child presents overlapping symptoms. If you suspect PANS or PANDAS and your family physician has no experience with it or will not consider it as a possible diagnosis, there is a network of physicians with expertise on PANS and PANDAS. This list can be found at pandasppn.org.

LYME DISEASE AND YOUR PETS

Your pets, whether they're wandering around in your yard, walking along a trail in the forest or running through long grass, are like tick magnets. During tick season (mainly spring and fall), my dog will have ticks crawling on her even after just a few minutes outside in the yard for a bathroom break. Fortunately, you have several tools in your tool kit to protect your pets from Lyme disease and OTBDs.

Dogs

Some might argue that dogs have it way better than humans when it comes to protection from Lyme and OTBDs. There is a vaccine that can be given to dogs to help prevent infection by *Borrelia* bacteria. When I adopted my puppy, she was about 16 weeks old. She received an initial Lyme vaccine, which was eventually followed by a booster shot. She will receive the Lyme vaccine annually. Your veterinarian can advise you on what age your dog needs to be vaccinated and on the frequency of the booster shots.

The Lyme vaccine is about 80 percent effective, so it is not perfect, and your dog could still contract Lyme disease despite being vaccinated (LaFleur et al. 2010). I strongly encourage you to do your homework to understand the pros and cons of the Lyme vaccine for your dog and to talk to your veterinarian about it. They are the experts when it comes to your pet's health. I know some

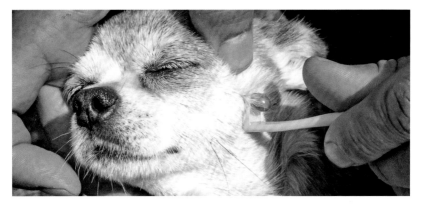

Frequent and thorough tick checks and early removal of found ticks are still the best ways to protect your four-legged friend.

people are concerned about overvaccinating their dogs. However, the effects of Lyme can be lethal, and the vaccine offers a very good level of protection against the disease.

In addition to the Lyme vaccine, various preventative treatments can be given to your dog to further protect them. I give my dog a product called NexGard, a beef-flavored treat that contains afoxolaner, an insecticide and acaricide that kills fleas and ticks. When consumed by your dog, the active ingredient circulates through your dog's bloodstream, and when your dog is bitten by a tick, that tick dies. I recently pulled an embedded tick that was plugged into my dog's head. The tick was dead, but it had clearly started feeding. Let's hope that what little feeding it did wasn't enough to transmit *Borrelia* bacteria (or any other microbes) to my dog and that the Lyme vaccine is helping to protect her too.

Where I live, the ticks are really active from March until mid-June and again from September until the end of November, so I use a flea and tick treatment on my dog from the end of February until the end of November. In areas with milder winters, dogs would likely need to be on a flea and tick treatment all year long. Consult your veterinarian to learn more about the products available and which ones they recommend for your pet.

Even though there are vaccines and monthly preventative treatments for dogs, it is still important to get any ticks off your dog as soon as possible — ideally before the ticks start feeding. Any feeding that a tick does presents an opportunity for it to transmit its microbes to your dog. Since the vaccine is 80 percent effective, doing tick checks on your dog after every foray outside is critical. Check all over. Ticks like to feed where the skin is thin and where there are lots of tiny blood vessels, so be sure to closely check your dog's face, ears, belly, legs, paws and between its toes. I find ticks hard to spot in the long fur on my dog's back but pretty easy to spot on her legs and face.

If your dog was bitten by a tick and you are worried about it contracting Lyme disease or OTBDs, there are tests your veterinarian can do to detect the presence of these infections. Single tests often look for multiple infections, such as Lyme, anaplasmosis, ehrlichiosis and heartworm. Like the tests for humans, these tests measure levels of antibodies. Talk to your veterinarian about testing if you are concerned about your dog's risk of contracting any of these infections.

In addition to having your dog tested for the presence of tick-borne infections, if you live in an area where ticks are abundant, it is also prudent to be aware of the symptoms of Lyme disease in dogs. Even if you take precautions, your dog can still contract the disease. If that happens, early detection and treatment are critical. The most common symptoms include fever, loss of appetite, painful or swollen joints and lameness, swollen lymph nodes and lethargy. However, some dogs show no symptoms. It is very important to treat Lyme disease in dogs early. If left untreated it can lead to kidney failure or damage to the heart or nervous system.

Cats

Until recently, it was thought that cats could not contract Lyme disease. However, recent research indicates that they can contract it, but that clinical disease is far more rare in cats than in dogs

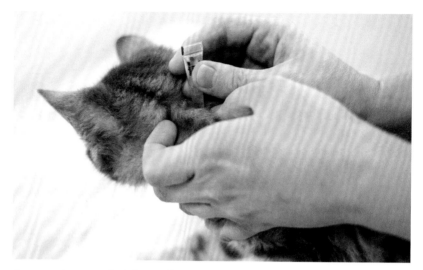

A cat receives a topical flea and tick treatment on the back of its neck.

(Tornqvist-Johnsen et al. 2020). My two cats stay indoors, but they do go out onto my screened porch. Mice and chipmunks occasionally sneak onto the porch and can bring ticks with them, which then drop off and attach onto the cats. If your cat is not being given a preventative treatment, then any ticks they bring into the house could also end up on you, which is how I think I ended up with a fully engorged tick on my back in 2019.

During the height of tick season, I treat my cats with a product called Bravecto. The active ingredient, fluralaner, is an insecticide and acaricide that kills fleas, ticks and some internal parasites. This particular product is a topical liquid that is applied to the skin on the back of a cat's neck, where the cat cannot lick it. As with treatment for a dog, talk to your veterinarian about the best option for protecting your cat, especially if it goes outdoors.

MOLD INFECTIONS

Mold infections can be another significant factor that contributes to the inflammation and multisystem disease caused by chronic Lyme. Anyone seeking a diagnosis of chronic Lyme disease

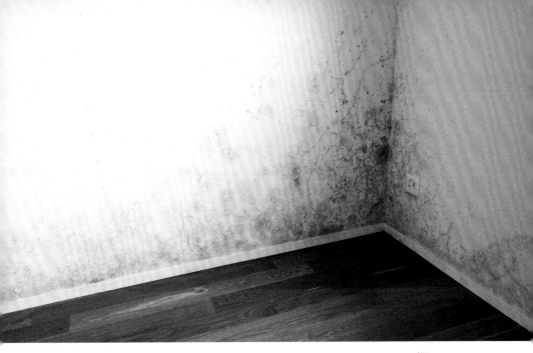

Black mold is most likely to appear in places with high cellulose content (fiber-board, gypsum board, drywall paper) that are humid, damp or water-damaged.

should also consider the possible involvement of molds. Molds make toxins called mycotoxins, which can enter your body in a number of ways: inhalation of mold hyphae (filaments) or spores (reproductive structures), absorption of mycotoxins through your skin, ingestion of hyphae, spores or mycotoxins through foods you eat, or exposure from mold already growing in your body (such as those molds that cause chronic sinus problems). Black mold is one of the biggest offenders when it comes to the effects of mycotoxins on our health. Inhalation of mold hyphae and spores occurs commonly from living in a house where mold is growing. Mold is especially problematic in older buildings or buildings where water damage has occurred and has not been

A great resource for understanding mold toxicity, especially in the context of Lyme disease, is Dr. Neil Nathan's 2018 book *Toxic: Heal Your Body from Mold Toxicity, Lyme Disease, Multiple Chemical Sensitivities, and Chronic Environmental Illness.*

dealt with adequately. Symptoms of mycotoxin exposure can include headaches, wheezing or trouble breathing, a sensation of electric shocks over the body, depression, anxiety and obsessive-compulsive thoughts and behaviors.

Why are mycotoxins so bad, and what do they have to do with Lyme disease? Mycotoxins cause inflammation and disrupt immune function (Nathan 2018). For example, ochratoxins, a type of mycotoxin you can be exposed to from water-damaged buildings and through ingesting contaminated foods, are known to cause kidney damage and cancer (Bui-Klimke and Wu 2015). According to the Great Plains Laboratory website, these mycotoxins can also cause oxidative damage to the brain and may contribute to neurodegenerative diseases such as Parkinson's and Alzheimer's. Ochratoxins can severely suppress the immune system, and their presence may contribute, through immune dysfunction, to the lack of antibodies produced in response to an infection with *Borrelia* bacteria or other tick-borne microbes. Other mycotoxins, such as mycophenolic acid, can also suppress the immune system. This suppression of the immune system then opens the door for coinfections with OTBDs.

In my case, it is likely that I had a latent *Borrelia* infection, which my immune system was able to keep in check before possibly becoming weakened from exposure to immune-suppressing mycotoxins, allowing the latent infection to emerge. The presence of mycotoxins can explain some of the symptoms we also see with Lyme disease and OTBDs, such as fatigue, headache, tingling and numbness, joint pain, shortness of breath and coughing, cognitive impairment and sensations of small electrical shocks all over the body.

The impacts mycotoxins have on the body are complex. As with Lyme disease, your family doctor will likely know little about mold toxicity or its potential role in chronic Lyme disease. This is why it is critical to find a Lyme-literate doctor who can help you.

Biofilms

Potentially important factors in chronic Lyme disease and OTBDs are biofilms. It is thought that biofilms may explain how infections can persist within the body and how the microbes avoid the effects of antibiotics used to treat Lyme disease.

Biofilms are aggregates of bacteria and other microbes (such as viruses, protozoa and fungi) that adhere to each other and form colonies. They typically secrete a slimy substance called a matrix that surrounds the microbial colony and forms a protective layer. This protective layer can prevent antibiotics from reaching the microbes and killing them, thus contributing to the persistence of infections. Once the protective layer of the biofilm forms, the community of microbes in that biofilm begin to function as a single cooperative unit (Rawls 2017) in which different microbes take on specialized roles, helping the entire colony to survive and thrive.

An example of a common biofilm is dental plaque (Marsh 2004). That coating on your teeth is actually a colony of different microbes that thrive in your mouth environment. Other biofilms that can cause harm to the body include bacterial vaginosis, chronic urinary tract infections, chronic sinusitis, chronic bronchitis, middle ear infections and arterial plaque (Rawls 2017). Not all biofilms are bad, however; there are protective biofilms that line your intestinal tract and help it to function properly. Biofilms that can do harm tend to form when your immune system is not functioning properly. There is still much more to learn about biofilms and Lyme.

COINFECTIONS

When you are bitten by a tick, it is highly likely that you are being infected with more than just Lyme bacteria. What you are infected with depends in part on where you live, but the important point to understand is that ticks are vectors of many different microbes. Worldwide, thousands of different microbes use ticks as an intermediate host (a host that transmits the microbe to its final host, typically a mammal). In North America, several diseases can result from a tick bite. Some of these coinfections are more common than others, although climate change is resulting in the northward movement of many of the microbes that cause these diseases (Pfeiffer 2018).

Having multiple tick-borne infections can make you much sicker than having only one. Some of these microbes produce effects and symptoms similar to those of Lyme disease, whereas others will contribute to different symptoms and affect different organs. All of these infections can contribute to immune dysfunction and multisystem inflammation. Chronic Lyme disease is notoriously difficult to treat effectively. The presence of other coinfections can hamper efforts to kill the *Borrelia* bacteria, reduce inflammation and resolve autoimmune issues. It usually means that a broader range of treatments is needed and that the treatment overall may take considerably longer.

Below is an overview of the most common tick-borne diseases in North America. Consult the resources listed in this book for more information on these tick-borne coinfections.

Babesiosis

Babesia is a piroplasm, a protozoan (single-celled) parasite in the order Piroplasmida. *Babesia* is an organism that has adapted to living in the cells and tissues of other animals. This parasite is transmitted by ticks, and it invades red blood cells in much the same way that the malaria parasite does, causing the blood cells to rupture. Given that red blood cells contain hemoglobin, which carries oxygen to your body's tissues, by attacking your red blood cells, *Babesia* reduces the transport of oxygen throughout your body. There are two species of *Babesia* known to occur in North America that infect humans: *Babesia microti* and *Babesia duncani* (the latter of which occurs primarily in western North America). Two species are currently known to occur in Europe: *Babesia divergens* and *Babesia venatorum*.

Hallmark symptoms of babesiosis (the name of the disease caused by a *Babesia* infection) include day sweats, drenching

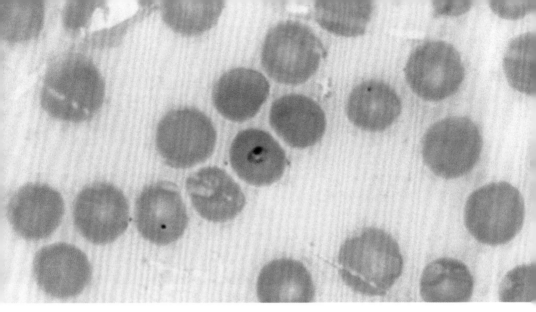

This photomicrograph of human blood shows *Babesia microti* in its young, ring stage.

night sweats, chills, flushing, cough, air hunger (an unexplained shortness of breath), fatigue and headache. It may also cause reduced appetite; fever; sleep disruption; muscle and joint aches; nausea or vomiting; balance problems; itching; sensations of pain, numbness or burning; sensitivity to light and sound; tinnitus (ear ringing); vertigo; and blurred vision. *Babesia* can affect the liver and spleen, resulting in an enlarged liver, enlarged spleen, jaundice (yellowing of the skin and whites of the eyes), enlarged lymph nodes and gastrointestinal problems. The infection is also known to cause marked psychological and psychiatric effects, such as short-term memory loss, problems concentrating, brain fog, anxiety, depression and mood swings. The symptoms of babesiosis may vary depending on the strain with which a person is infected (Horowitz 2013).

Most doctors in North America have little to no knowledge of babesiosis, including its symptoms, how to diagnose it and how to treat it. I have encountered physicians who base their understanding of the prevalence of *Babesia* on its detection in blood donation products — a statistic that is not indicative of the number of ticks or people infected with the parasite.

Like Lyme disease, babesiosis can persist for years as a latent infection with no obvious symptoms, but when the immune system ceases to function well, the latent infection can become active, causing symptoms. Babesiosis can be a dangerous illness, and in some cases, it can cause death. It is the second-most common tick-borne infection in North America; the proportion of people infected with Lyme who are also infected with *Babesia* can be as high as 65 percent (Schaller 2006).

As with Lyme disease, testing for babesiosis is notoriously unreliable (Horowitz 2013) and generally depends on the presence of antibodies or on direct observation of infected red blood cells examined under a microscope. As with Lyme disease, a negative test result doesn't necessarily mean you are not infected with the parasite. Like malaria, babesiosis is typically treated with a course of antimalarial medication, often combined with the antibiotic azithromycin.

Bartonellosis

Bartonella is a bacterium that can be transmitted through a tick bite. It is thought to occur in 25 percent to 50 percent of patients with Lyme disease (Rawls 2017). *Bartonella* bacteria cause bartonellosis, which is also called cat-scratch disease — so named because it can also be transmitted through a scratch from a domestic or feral cat. (Cats can become infected from the bite of an infected flea or louse.) It is thought that *Bartonella* can also be transmitted through the bites of sand flies or mosquitoes (Nathan 2018). In North America, *Bartonella henselae* is the main species that results in tick-borne bartonellosis, although other species are known.

Bartonella infects the body's endothelial cells, which are the cells that line your blood vessels (Rawls 2017). Like *Borrelia* bacteria, *Bartonella* are able to hide in the body by leaving the bloodstream and living in a variety of organs (e.g., liver, kidney, brain) where they can evade the immune system and antibiotic treatments (Scherler et al. 2018). *Bartonella* can affect multiple organs, such as the liver, spleen, eyes, skin, bone marrow, heart and other parts of the vascular system (related to arteries and veins), causing symptoms such as a rash (consisting of raised red bumps), malaise, headache, fatigue, swollen lymph nodes, sore throat, joint and muscle pain, gastrointestinal issues, pelvic pain and eye issues. Two of the hallmark symptoms of bartonellosis are painful, burning sensations on the bottoms of the feet and the presence of red lines on the body that look like stretch marks. Like Lyme and babesiosis, bartonellosis can also cause neurological and psychiatric symptoms such as anxiety, depression, extreme mood swings (including feelings of rage, another hallmark of bartonellosis), Bell's palsy (facial paralysis) and numbing or tingling sensations. It can also cause a sensation of trembling or vibration throughout the entire body. I have experienced this, and I described to my doctor that it felt as if my entire body was vibrating, with the vibrations originating from deep within. Dr. Neil Nathan indicates that the neurological symptoms of bartonellosis may overlap with those of atypical MS, Parkinson's disease, Alzheimer's disease and ALS (Nathan 2018). A blood test is used to detect bartonellosis. As with Lyme and *Babesia*, the *Bartonella* test often fails to detect the bacteria or yields inconclusive results, so a negative test result does not necessarily mean you do not have bartonellosis. Because *Bartonella* is a bacterium, it is treated with antibiotics.

Ehrlichiosis

Ehrlichia is a type of bacterium that causes a disease called ehrlichiosis. There are several species that can infect humans, and they are transmitted by *Ixodes scapularis*, the black-legged tick. However, the bacterium that causes human monocytic ehrlichiosis is transmitted specifically by the lone star tick. Common symptoms of ehrlichiosis include flu-like symptoms, such as a high fever, severe headache, malaise, fatigue and muscle pain. Although ehrlichiosis is thought of as a less-common tick-borne infection in North America, a study by Evason et al. in 2019 recorded a 150 percent increase in the prevalence of *Ehrlichia* bacteria in dogs between 2008 and 2015.

Ehrlichiosis is a nasty disease that should be taken seriously and treated immediately as it can be fatal for individuals with a compromised immune system. As with all tick-borne infections, clinical diagnosis is essential but should be accompanied by blood tests to support the diagnosis. Like for Lyme disease, the blood test for ehrlichiosis detects antibodies; however, physicians can also look for evidence of an infection through common blood tests, such as a complete blood count. Abnormalities such as a low white blood cell count, low platelet count and elevated liver enzymes (AST and ALT) can help with diagnosis. Because *Ehrlichia* is a bacterium, it is treated with antibiotics.

Anaplasmosis

Anaplasmosis is caused by a bacterial infection. There are several species of bacteria that cause anaplasmosis, but *Anaplasma phagocytophilum* is the most common cause in North America. Symptoms include flu-like symptoms, such as a high fever and muscle pain, as well as nausea, vomiting, diarrhea and loss of appetite. If left untreated, anaplasmosis, like other tick-borne infections, can be life-threatening. As with ehrlichiosis, the diagnosis should be based on a clinical diagnosis supported by blood tests. Antibiotics are used to treat this bacterial infection.

Rocky Mountain Spotted Fever

Rickettsia rickettsii is the species of bacteria that causes Rocky Mountain spotted fever (RMSF). Related species — *Rickettsia typhi* and *Coxiella burnetii* — cause typhus and Q fever, respectively. RMSF can be transmitted by the black-legged tick as well as the Rocky Mountain wood tick, American dog tick, brown dog tick and lone star tick. Symptoms include fever, nausea, vomiting, headache, muscle pain and other flu-like symptoms. RMSF can also cause red spots on wrists, forearms, ankles, palms of hands and soles of feet, although this rash is highly variable and is not always present. The illness can be fatal in up to 10 percent of cases if left untreated, especially in the very young, very old and those with a compromised immune system (Nelder et al. 2020). It is one of the most dangerous tick-borne infections in North America and should be taken very seriously.

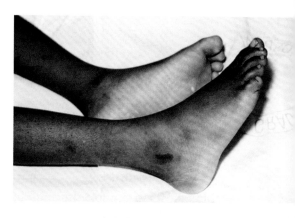
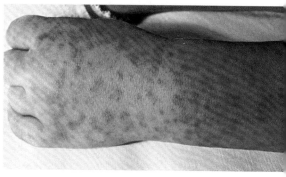

These photos show types of rashes caused by RMSF.

As with ehrlichiosis and anaplasmosis, blood tests can be used to aid in the diagnosis. Abnormalities such as a low white blood cell count, low platelet count and elevated liver enzymes (AST and ALT) are often seen with this disease. RMSF is treated with antibiotics.

Mycoplasmosis

Mycoplasma is a type of bacterium that infects white blood cells and causes a disease called mycoplasmosis. Like *Borrelia*, *Mycoplasma* can hide out in the joints and brain, and also like *Borrelia*, it manipulates the immune system and causes inflammation. About three-quarters of those with chronic Lyme are also thought to have mycoplasmosis (Rawls 2017). Symptoms of mycoplasmosis include flu-like symptoms, such as muscle pain, fatigue and joint pain. Blood tests for mycoplasmosis are unreliable and given the overlap of symptoms with diseases like Lyme, it can be difficult to diagnose. Because it is a bacterial infection, mycoplasmosis is treated with antibiotics. However, like chronic Lyme disease, mycoplasmosis can be difficult to eradicate and may require long-term treatment.

Powassan Virus

Powassan virus is a tick-borne infection that is currently considered quite rare, but there is concern that the disease may become more prevalent. Powassan virus has been detected in ticks in eastern and central North America. Symptoms of the disease include fever, seizures and inflammation of the brain, which can cause neurological symptoms such as changes to vision, hearing and mental status, as well as hemiplegia (paralysis of one-half of the body) and loss of consciousness. Chronic effects can result in the inability to walk. Powassan virus can be fatal in up to 10 percent of cases in which severe neurological symptoms are present. Tests for the virus are done by detecting antibodies in either blood or cerebrospinal fluid. There is currently no known treatment for the disease, aside from supportive measures, such as hospitalization, respiratory support and intravenous fluids to help reduce symptoms. According to Dr. Richard Horowitz, a Lyme-literate medical doctor in the United States with years of experience treating Lyme disease and OTBDs, the virus can be transmitted within as little as 15 minutes of a tick bite (Horowitz 2013). This is another reason why it is so important to take precautions against possible tick bites and to remove any biting ticks immediately.

Southern Tick-Associated Rash Illness

As with RMSF, southern tick-associated rash illness (STARI) is transmitted by the lone star tick. It causes Lyme-like flu symptoms, including fever, headache, fatigue, muscle ache and joint pain. The disease can also produce a bull's-eye rash.

Because the exact cause of STARI is still unknown, no blood tests exist yet that can aid in diagnosis of the disease. Instead, diagnosis relies only on clinical symptoms and geographic location, since the disease occurs primarily in southeastern and south-central United States. However, the range of the lone star tick, and its corresponding infections, is expanding. From 2017 to 2019, nine lone star ticks were reported by the

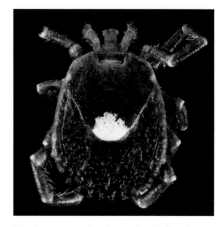

The lone star tick is gradually finding its way north and may become more of an issue in the northeastern United States and Canada.

Wellington-Dufferin-Guelph Public Health Unit in Ontario, and in 2019, a lone star tick was discovered on a cat in London, Ontario. This tick species is also responsible for ehrlichiosis, Heartland virus and Bourbon virus, and its saliva is known to contain a carbohydrate called alpha-gal, which triggers an antibody response and results in an anaphylactic reaction to red meat (beef, lamb, pork and other mammals) and mammal-derived products, such as milk and gelatin.

A number of other diseases in North America are transmitted by ticks, and this book focuses on the most prevalent ones. Although the diseases discussed here are the most common tick-borne diseases in North America, your family doctor will likely have little to no knowledge of them or how to diagnose and treat them. Therefore, you should seek help from a Lyme-literate doctor who is familiar with the symptoms and the likelihood of the various coinfections and who will know how to treat them. Consulting a Lyme-literate doctor is also important because, as with *Borrelia*, testing for many of these coinfections is notoriously poor. Although serologic testing can be done for most, these test results can be unreliable, and a clinical diagnosis should always be conducted.

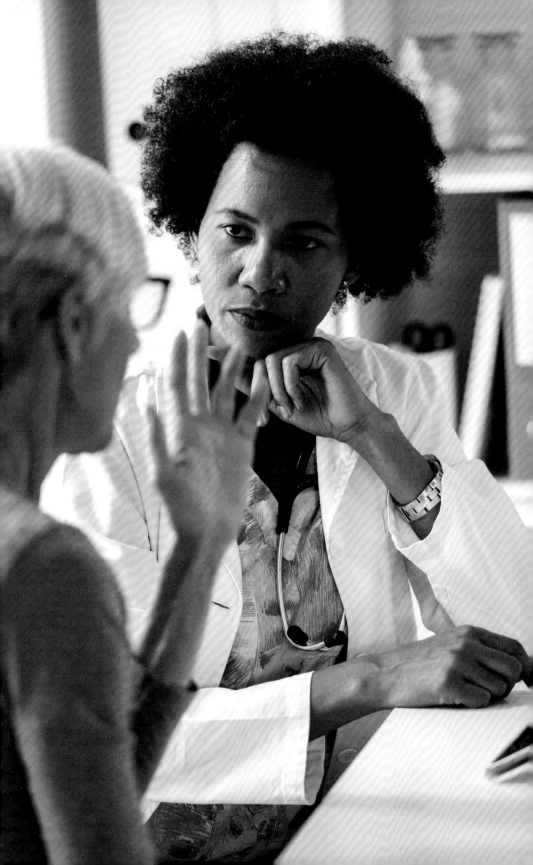

CHAPTER **5**

Diagnosing Lyme Disease

Diagnosing Lyme disease is currently a very controversial topic and there are divergent views on how it should be done. It is not straightforward, in that a simple serologic test (a blood test that looks for antibodies) all too often cannot provide a definitive answer. The most important point to understand here is that a diagnosis of Lyme disease should be based on a *clinical diagnosis*, one that considers symptoms and other factors, such as the patient's history, activity and location. Blood tests can be used to support a diagnosis, but they should not be relied on to make a diagnosis due to their poor performance.

CLINICAL DIAGNOSIS

A clinical diagnosis takes into account a patient's history, where they live (in other words, do they live in a Lyme hot spot?), risk factors, symptoms and other clinical findings.

A patient's history includes whether they've found a tick on their body, saw only a bite mark (but no tick) or had no idea

◄ A clinical diagnosis of Lyme, which factors in symptoms, history, activity and location, is crucial where serologic testing fails.

The Horowitz Lyme Multiple Systemic Infectious Disease Syndrome Questionnaire

Because of the broad range of symptoms Lyme disease and OTBDs have and their overlap with those of other diseases and conditions, you should look at the entire range of symptoms you experience after your tick bite. This includes noting the *severity* of your symptoms and *when* they show up. To aid in diagnosis, Dr. Richard Horowitz developed a checklist of symptoms, compiled as the Horowitz Lyme Multiple Systemic Infectious Disease Syndrome Questionnaire, to help determine the likelihood of Lyme disease. A person fills out the questionnaire and scores the symptoms based on their severity. There are four sections in the questionnaire, and at the end, the total scores of each section are added to produce an overall score.

- A score of 46 or more means that there is a high probability that Lyme disease is involved; you should seek the help of a Lyme-literate doctor for diagnosis.
- A score of 21 to 45 means Lyme disease may be involved; you may consider seeking help from a Lyme-literate doctor.
- A score of under 21 means Lyme is unlikely to be the cause of your symptoms.

For example, when I was at my sickest, my Horowitz score was 126. I had nearly every symptom, and each one was severe. At that point I was barely able to walk more than a few steps. The Horowitz questionnaire and the diary I used to track my daily symptoms (see page 79) were instrumental in my clinical diagnosis of Lyme disease.

Completing the questionnaire and bringing it to your doctor's appointment with your symptom diary may greatly help your doctor in making a diagnosis. Scan the QR code or visit this site to download the questionnaire: cangetbetter.com/wp-content /uploads/2020/11/BLP_MISIDS LymeQuestionnaire.pdf

that they were bitten by a tick. Often a patient never sees the tick because they don't feel it biting them, and the tick drops off before it is detected. As we learned in Chapter 2, tick nymphs are so small that they may go undetected or be mistaken for a speck of dirt. If the patient never found a tick on them nor noticed a bite, then it is especially important to understand that their risk of a tick bite should be based on where they live and on their activities.

If a patient lives in or has traveled to a region where Lyme disease is endemic (known to be well established in the tick population), then the risk of Lyme is substantial, and this should be a major consideration in the diagnosis. If a patient has a job that requires them to spend a lot of time outdoors (for example, farmers, arborists, landscapers, field biologists and so on) or if they engage in activities that lead them to spend a lot of time out-doors in habitats where ticks live, then this, too, should factor into the diagnosis. Remember: Just because you didn't see the tick on you or didn't end up with a bull's-eye rash, it does not necessarily mean you do not have Lyme disease.

To understand the geographic variation in the risk of exposure to Lyme disease, many public health agencies provide maps that outline areas where there is a risk of contracting the disease. As an example, in 2016 the Government of Canada compiled data from the provincial health agencies to produce the map on page 118, which shows the areas of the country where people are most at risk of contracting Lyme.

You should note that the accuracy of these types of maps in reflecting the actual distribution of ticks and risk of Lyme disease may be questionable for a number of reasons. First, they depend on the case definition of Lyme disease, which also affects report-ing of the disease. For example, if a public health system does not recognize chronic Lyme disease, it will not report it. As a result, the number of cases of Lyme is likely underreported, particularly in Canada, and therefore, these types of maps should be inter-preted with this in mind. Second, you should understand that black-legged ticks and the risk of Lyme disease are not confined

Lyme Risk Areas in Canada in 2016
(risk areas are increasing)

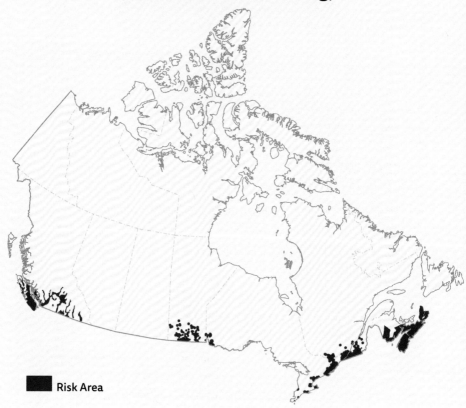

Risk Area

just to the areas defined on a map. Public Health Ontario, for example, states on its Lyme risk map, "Despite these estimated risk areas, it is important to note that blacklegged ticks feed on and are transported by migratory birds, meaning there is a possibility of encountering an infective blacklegged tick almost anywhere in Ontario." This is crucial information because, based on my own experiences and conversations with other Lyme sufferers, many health professionals will dismiss a Lyme diagnosis if they believe that Lyme disease is not an issue in the area. This is problematic because, as noted, there is insufficient data on the occurrence of Lyme disease across Canada and the United States,

Here are QR codes and links to Lyme disease risk maps in the United States and Canada:

Canada: www.canada.ca/en/public-health/services/diseases /lyme-disease/risk-lyme-disease.html

United States: www.cdc.gov/lyme/datasurveillance/maps -recent.html

Note: Your particular province/state or county might have more specific information on their public health website.

and the risk of contracting Lyme increases every year as tick populations and their ranges grow. Ticks increase their range by about 16 miles (25 kilometers) per year, meaning that geographically, the area where Lyme disease has the potential to occur increases every year as well. Additionally, ticks that are carried on the bodies of migratory birds will be able to survive in any part of North America where the climate and habitat are favorable, so anyone in those locations potentially is at risk for the disease. In short, these types of maps should not be used to determine whether treatment for Lyme is warranted or not.

All of these things — patient history, geography, other risk factors — along with symptoms, need to be considered in diagnosing Lyme.

DIAGNOSTIC TESTING

In the October 2012 bulletin of *Canadian Adverse Reaction Newsletter*, a publication directed at health professionals, Health Canada states that "serologic test results are supplemental to the clinical diagnosis of Lyme disease and should not be the primary basis for making diagnostic or treatment decisions." The bulletin further states, "Lyme disease test kits have sensitivity and specificity limitations.... Health care professionals should be aware of these limitations and are encouraged to report suspected incidents, including false-positive and false-negative results, to Health Canada."

In other words, the Government of Canada has advised health professionals to rely on clinical diagnosis and that serologic tests are only supplemental to the clinical diagnosis. Despite this, most health professionals in Canada and far too many, still, in the

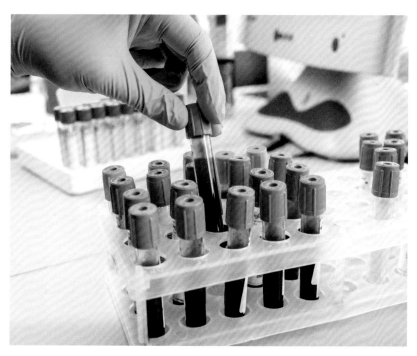

Serologic tests for Lyme can be unreliable and yet many doctors rely on the test results in their diagnosis.

United States rely primarily and often solely on the results of sero-logic testing or on the presence of a bull's-eye rash to diagnose Lyme disease. As a result, many, many cases of Lyme disease are being missed and the number of North Americans left untreated and who go on to develop late disseminated and chronic Lyme is unacceptably large. It should be noted, though, that the United States seems to have more accurate case reporting than Canada.

One of the most important things to understand about serologic testing for Lyme disease is that *a negative Lyme test does not necessarily mean you don't have Lyme disease*. While it can certainly mean that you do not *have* antibodies to the Lyme bacteria in your body, it can also mean the test failed to detect those antibodies, which would be the case if the test were done shortly after the infection, when antibody levels are low, or late in the infection, when the immune system is no longer making antibodies for the Lyme bacteria. Unfortunately, the test cannot distinguish between these two possibilities, yet most doctors insist on interpreting a negative test as meaning that the patient does not have Lyme disease, despite strong clinical support for a Lyme diagnosis. So if you exhibit the symptoms of Lyme disease, have spent time outside where ticks live and, therefore, could have been bitten by a tick, then your symptoms and risk of infection by Lyme bacteria should be the criteria used to make a diagnosis. If you know you were bitten by a tick (i.e., you saw the tick on you and removed it) and you have the symptoms of Lyme disease, but your serologic test comes back negative, *the result of the test alone should not be used to determine your course of treatment*. Ignoring the symptoms could lead to chronic Lyme disease, which is difficult and sometimes impossible to cure.

Types of Tests

Several types of tests are used to detect Lyme disease, each with its own advantages and disadvantages. In this section, we will explore some of the more common tests used in North America.

You should note that many of these tests may not be covered by your public health care system or your insurance, and they might require out-of-pocket payment.

Two-Tier Testing

Antibodies are proteins that a healthy immune system creates to fight foreign invaders, such as bacteria and viruses, that enter your body. They do this by binding to antigens, which are substances (usually proteins) on the surface of the foreign substances. The antibody either directly neutralizes the foreign substance or flags it for other parts of the immune system to attack.

There are several types of antibodies, but two we will discuss are immunoglobulin M (IgM) and immunoglobulin G (IgG). IgM antibodies are present in the blood early on in an infection, while IgG antibodies, which are the most common, can take a while to form and are usually interpreted as an indicator of past infection.

Serologic tests try to detect antibodies in a blood sample, so a Lyme test essentially tests for whether your body has had to fight an infection caused by Lyme bacteria.

Many public health care systems typically use a two-tier approach to serologic testing for Lyme disease. This means that potentially two different antibody tests would be done to look for evidence of a Lyme infection. When your doctor does a Lyme test, they draw your blood and send it away to a laboratory for testing, and you typically receive your test results within a week.

The first of the two types of tests administered is called an enzyme-linked immunosorbent assay (ELISA). This test looks for antibodies, the proteins made by your immune system that bind to antigens on the Lyme bacteria. As I will discuss starting on page 127, there are a number of reasons why you can have Lyme disease and yet negative ELISA test results — something that will be crucial for your doctor to understand. Note that ELISA yields a

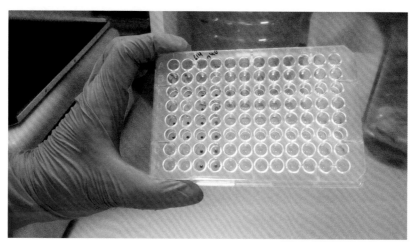

A lab technician holds a typical ELISA test plate.

qualitative test result that is either positive or negative. The test provides no other information for interpretation.

With two-tier testing, if the initial ELISA test is negative, a second (confirmatory) test is often done about 30 days later. The reason for this is that the ELISA test lacks sensitivity. If the test is done too soon after a tick bite, your immune system may not have had enough time to produce enough antibodies for the test to detect them. By retesting a month later, it allows more time for the body to generate the antibodies.

The second part of the two-tier approach is called a Western blot (or an immunoblot). This test is only done if the first test, ELISA (which is a much less sensitive test), is positive. A Western blot looks at whether antibodies in the patient's blood attach to various antigens isolated from Lyme bacteria. An electric current is applied to a medium on which these antigens sit. The electric current causes the antigens to move, with smaller ones moving farther than the larger ones. This results in various antigens being sorted by molecular weight (measured in kilodaltons [kDa]) and that produce visible band patterns. With IgM antibodies, two of three significant bands must be present for the test to be considered positive (Canadian Public Health Laboratory Network 2007; CDC 1995). With IgG antibodies, five of 10 significant bands must be present for the test to be considered positive. The problem with this approach is that people with Lyme disease who display severe symptoms may have fewer than five bands present. Furthermore, CDC removed two bands (the 31 kDa and 34 kDa bands) from the diagnostic criteria for the Western blot. The two bands removed are very specific to Lyme disease and yet they were excluded because they were used to create a Lyme disease vaccine, and anyone who received it would presumably test positive for those two bands. To facilitate the manufacture of a negative Lyme test for those who had received the vaccine, CDC decided to remove those two bands despite their being highly specific to Lyme disease. The vaccine was discontinued in 2002 due to its ineffectiveness, *yet these two*

Lyme Testing and Gender

Gender might play a role in receiving an accurate Lyme diagnosis. Women may be less likely to receive a diagnosis when they have Lyme disease, and they may experience a higher incidence of treatment failure.

In commercial two-tier Lyme testing, men are more likely to test positive with ELISA and Western blot tests (Rebman et al. 2015; Schwarzwalder et al. 2010). As noted for the Western blot, CDC requires that five of 10 bands be present for the test to be considered positive. Men tend to have six positive bands, and women tend to have four positive bands. Therefore, women may be less likely to test positive for Lyme and receive timely diagnosis and treatment compared to men (Stricker and Johnson 2009).

This is alarming because research has shown women may be more likely to be bitten by a tick because they attract more ticks, and they present more atypical Lyme rashes. Women also tend to produce more inflammatory and inhibitory cytokines than men (Jarefors 2006).

More research is needed to better understand gender differences in the diagnosis and treatment of Lyme, but this is something to keep in mind.

important bands continue to be excluded from interpretation of Western blot tests, resulting in many cases of Lyme disease going undiagnosed.

The Western blot is a more comprehensive test than ELISA in that it is more sensitive and can detect the presence of lower numbers of antibodies to *Borrelia* (which generally occurs in both early- and late-stage Lyme), but doctors only conduct the Western blot as a confirmatory test if the ELISA test is positive. This is problematic because it means that the less accurate test, which results in far too many false-negative results, is used to determine whether the more comprehensive test is done. The Western blot is not without its own problems; however, it is still the better of the two tests and yet remains underused in assisting with a Lyme diagnosis.

A meta-analysis (Cook and Puri 2016) that surveyed the results of studies published in peer-reviewed science journals showed how poorly two-tier testing for Lyme disease performs. The results indicated that using the two-tier approach, the tests were negative even though patients did have Lyme disease 54.7 percent of the time. This is why overreliance on serologic testing leads to many missed cases of Lyme disease.

IGeneX Lyme Immunoblot

A variety of other Lyme tests can be ordered from private laboratories. In most cases you have to pay for these out of your own pocket, but it may be worth doing if you are struggling to get a clinical diagnosis from your doctor.

There is a newer immunoblot test offered by a lab called IGeneX that uses synthetic proteins created from recombinant DNA (using DNA strands from different strains that have been combined). The test uses only proteins that are specific to Lyme disease, which reduces the chances of a false-positive result. For the IgM antibodies, this test is considered positive if it produces bands at two or more of the following five proteins: 23 kDa, 31 kDa, 34 kDa, 39 kDa and 41 kDa. For the IgG antibodies, a test is considered positive if it produces bands at two of the following five proteins: 23 kDa, 31 kDa, 34 kDa, 39 kDa and 93 kDa.

Another advantage of the immunoblot test from IGeneX is that it tests for eight strains of Lyme proteins: *B. burgdorferi* B31, *B. burgdorferi* 297, *B. californiensis*, *B. mayonii*, *B. spielmanii*, *B. afzelii*, *B. garinii* and *B. valaisiana*.

Polymerase Chain Reaction

A polymerase chain reaction (PCR) is a test that looks for the presence of *Borrelia* DNA rather than the presence of antibodies that a person's immune system may manufacture in response to *Borrelia*. Although this sounds like a more direct approach to detecting Lyme, it also has its limitations. PCR of blood samples will only detect bacteria if they are in the bloodstream. *Borrelia* bacteria do not remain in the bloodstream for long, so the timing of the test matters. Lyme bacteria do not like oxygen-rich environments like blood, so they invade the oxygen-poor tissues with limited blood flow, such as joints, tendons, ligaments and fascia (the fibrous covering of muscle tissue). It is possible to attempt to sample these tissues for PCR analysis; however, obtaining a sufficient sample

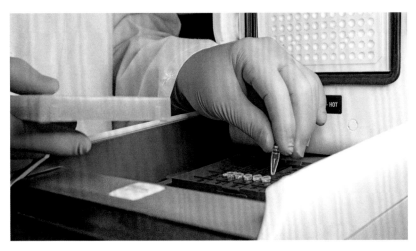

A technician loads PCR tubes into a thermal cycler.

can be an invasive procedure, with no guarantee of detection. Furthermore, there is no way to know the exact location of the bacteria, so sampling tissue to look for *Borrelia* DNA can be like looking for a needle in a haystack. PCR of urine samples has also been used as a detection method because *Borrelia* bacteria are excreted in urine, but there are studies showing that this is not a reliable way of detecting the bacterium (Rauter et al. 2005).

EliSpot

Another test called an enzyme-linked immunosorbent spot (EliSpot) detects whether T cells (a type of immune cell) have been exposed to Lyme bacteria. T cells that have been exposed to antigens on the surface of Lyme bacteria produce a chemical called gamma interferon. The test is very sensitive and can pick up weaker immune responses to the presence of the Lyme bacteria.

This test can be done through IGeneX, California, or Armin Labs, Germany.

Why Are My Lyme Tests Negative?

So far I have written about some of the Lyme tests that are available. I've barely scratched the surface of this topic, and I recommend that you consult the Resources section on page 156 for more information and that you discuss it with your Lyme-literate doctor.

Regardless of the test, I can't emphasize enough that a negative Lyme test does not necessarily mean you don't have Lyme disease. False-negative test results are common with the two-tier Lyme testing approach.

Your family doctor or an ER doctor is unlikely to know much about Lyme disease, so it is critical for you to educate yourself and be prepared to advocate assertively for yourself and your own health care. For me, part of this involved understanding why my Lyme tests were negative despite having nearly every symptom of Lyme disease. These explanations for why my Lyme test could

Private Labs

IGenex, Armin Labs and other private labs offer various tests for Lyme disease. Consult a Lyme-literate doctor for guidance on which tests to order because the cost of testing at these labs may not be covered by your public health care system or any health insurance you have.

In the United States, doctors are more likely to accept test results from IGeneX, but a word of caution for Canadians: In my experience, both IGeneX and Armin Labs are reputable and perform validation tests to measure the reliability of their tests. However, most doctors in Canada will not accept or recognize test results from these private labs. They consider these labs biased and accuse them of generating high numbers of false-positive results. Testing with private labs should be done for your own information and for that of the Lyme-literate physician who is overseeing your health care.

When I was desperately sick with Lyme disease and OTBDs, knowing that I could obtain tests from private labs gave me hope. However, getting tests done at these labs was a battle. For tests done at IGeneX, a licensed doctor must provide authorization. Authorization from your family doctor might be impossible to obtain if they do not view private labs as producing valid results. Armin Labs does not require a doctor's authorization to have the tests done; however, I encountered another hurdle. In Ontario, you must have a requisition from an authorized health practitioner to have your blood drawn, even if you are willing to pay for the cost of the procedure out of your own pocket. While I eventually had a doctor authorize it, for a while it prevented me from accessing the private testing. For me this raised the question: Shouldn't I have the right to pay for the procedures that will give me the information necessary to help regain my health?

be negative were essential to me receiving a clinical diagnosis of Lyme disease that was based on my symptoms, history and risk of exposure to Lyme bacteria.

Here are the possible reasons why your test results (for any test, not just the serologic tests recommended by Health Canada and CDC) could be negative:

1. *You don't have Lyme disease:* This is always a possibility, but it is only one of several explanations for a negative test result. If you have a number of symptoms of Lyme disease, have spent time outdoors in habitats that ticks favor and you live or have visited an area where Lyme disease is prevalent, and yet you still tested negative, then you might consider trying a different type of test (other than the standard two-tier testing) and consulting a Lyme-literate doctor.

2. *You have Lyme disease, but you do not have sufficient antibody levels for the test to detect them:* Serologic tests depend on the presence of antibodies for Lyme bacteria in your bloodstream. It is well known that the ELISA test, the first of the two tests in the two-tier testing scheme, lacks sensitivity. This means that it is not very good at detecting antibodies for Lyme bacteria when they occur at low numbers. Antibodies for *Borrelia* can be low early on in the infection, not long after the bite, because your immune system hasn't had enough time to create enough antibodies for the test to detect them. This is also why a confirmatory ELISA test is usually done about 30 days after the first test. The logic behind this approach is that after 30 days your immune system should have produced enough antibodies to be detectable by the ELISA test. The problem with this approach is that there is only a narrow window of time (approximately two weeks) during which to treat Lyme with antibiotics and maximize the chance of killing the Lyme bacteria. Waiting longer than two weeks reduces the chance that antibiotic treatment will be effective. This is especially true if your doctor will only prescribe a short course (two to three weeks) of antibiotic treatment. Getting too short a course of antibiotics and receiving them too late can reduce the chances of killing a Lyme infection.

3. *You have Lyme disease, but there are no antibodies in your blood-stream for the test to detect:* As mentioned above, serologic tests depend on the presence of antibodies for Lyme bacteria. There are a few reasons why your immune system would not be manufacturing antibodies to *Borrelia* bacteria and, therefore, why there are no antibodies in your bloodstream for the test to detect. First, *Borrelia* bacteria remain in the bloodstream for a very short period of time (Liang et al. 2020). These bacteria do not like oxygen-rich environments, and the bloodstream is oxygen-rich, since one of the functions of blood is to deliver oxygen to the body's tissues. Instead, the bacteria hide out in low-oxygen environments, such as the joints. In the blood-stream, *Borrelia* bacteria typically exist in their spirochetal form, but when they exit the bloodstream and burrow into the tissues they can change into "persister" forms, such as round bodies. In this state, they can remain dormant (nonreproduc-ing) in the tissues for months or even years (Rudenko et al. 2019). When *Borrelia* bacteria lodge themselves into tissues and change to their round-body form, antibiotics have a difficult time reaching them, so antibiotic treatments are far less effec-tive during this stage of Lyme disease (Meriläinen et al. 2015).

The second reason why there may be no antibodies for *Borrelia* bacteria in your bloodstream is that *Borrelia* are "stealth" bacteria. In addition to their main strand of DNA, *Borrelia* bacteria have plasmids, which are extra bits of DNA that exist as short circular or linear strands. The bacteria are able to change their genetic makeup by shuffling their plasmid DNA. By doing this, they can change their surface proteins, which allows them to hide from your immune system. Your immune system looks for a specific type of surface protein to identify the "invader," the *Borrelia* bacterium, and makes antibodies based on this pro-tein, but if *Borrelia* changes its surface proteins it will fool your immune system into thinking that the bacterium is gone.

It is clear that the fascinating biology of *Borrelia* bacteria and the inadequate tests for detecting their presence contribute to the abundance of false-negative tests in patients who really do have Lyme disease. All of this reinforces the need for clinical diagnosis. Without it, far too many cases of Lyme disease will be missed and far too many people will end up with chronic Lyme, a disease that can be extremely debilitating and very difficult to cure.

Given the overreliance by medical professionals on the results of serologic testing for Lyme disease, and the lack of knowledge about Lyme disease by most family and ER doctors, it is important to understand that you will most likely need to become an assertive advocate for your own medical care or that of your loved ones. (If you are unable to advocate for yourself or your loved ones, find someone who is able to do this.) You may very well have to educate your doctor about the issues surrounding a Lyme disease diagnosis and persuade them to do a clinical diagnosis to determine whether you have Lyme disease. If you have the symptoms of Lyme disease, live in (or have visited) an area where black-legged ticks are found or where Lyme disease is known to occur, and you spend time outdoors in places where ticks may live, then a diagnosis of Lyme disease should be made and an appropriate course of treatment given. I have an excellent family doctor, but in my experience, it took me showing up to her office very ill and with a stack of peer-reviewed science journal articles about Lyme disease before I could convince her to rely on a clinical diagnosis rather than two negative serologic tests. In the end, she did a clinical diagnosis, and I am grateful for that. Unfortunately, the six weeks of antibiotic treatment I was prescribed wasn't enough to get me well again, so I had to seek other avenues of help. This also shows the importance of getting a diagnosis quickly: It took seven weeks to convince my doctor that what I was suffering from was Lyme disease, which meant that the early treatment window had passed.

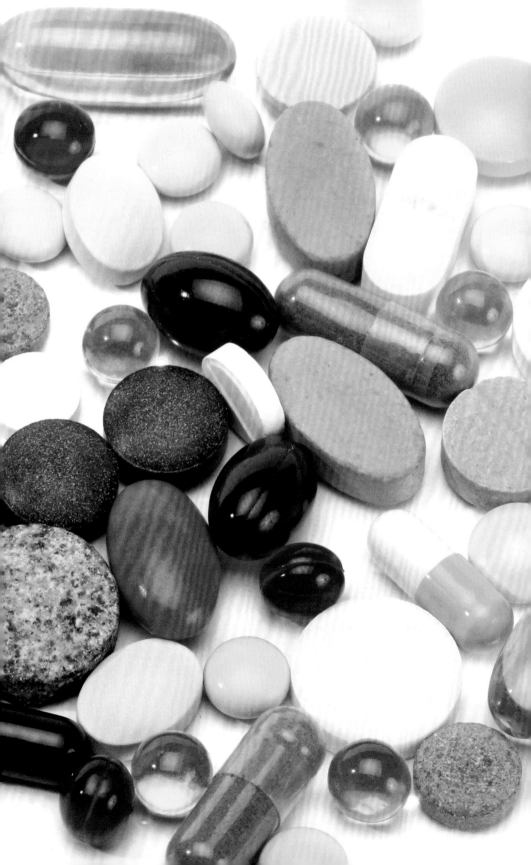

CHAPTER 6

Treating Lyme and Coinfections

If treated soon enough after a tick bite, Lyme disease can likely be eradicated with a sufficient course of antibiotic treatment. The International Lyme and Associated Diseases Society (ILADS) guidelines recommend four to six weeks of antibiotics (Cameron et al. 2014). However, many family doctors and ER doctors will not prescribe a course of antibiotics this long, especially if no bull's-eye rash was seen or if the patient tests negative with serologic testing. This results in undertreatment and the probable persistence of the infection, leading to chronic Lyme disease.

Another complication arises if your doctor follows the treatment guidelines of the Infectious Diseases Society of America (IDSA). The IDSA recommends a shorter course of antibiotics than ILADS — two to three weeks instead of four to six. While a shorter course of antibiotics may be enough to kill all the bacteria within the first few weeks of your bite, because of the difficulties a patient can face getting a Lyme diagnosis quickly, often the bacteria have already disseminated to the tissues and organs by the time Lyme

◄ Lyme treatment often combines prescription drugs with herbal medicines and lifestyle adjustments.

is suspected. At this point, 14 to 21 days of antibiotic treatment is highly unlikely to eradicate a *Borrelia* infection (or any other bacterial tick-borne infection), and once again, undertreatment and the possible persistence of infection can lead to chronic Lyme disease.

As discussed previously, chronic Lyme disease (along with OTBDs) results in an illness that can affect multiple organ systems. The combined impacts of the *Borrelia* bacteria and coinfections on the immune system lead to significant systemic inflammation. Therefore, treatment of chronic Lyme needs to be focused not just on killing the Lyme bacteria and coinfections, but also on reducing systemic inflammation and building the immune system back up.

There are excellent books written entirely about treating Lyme disease that will give you a deep dive into treatment approaches and options, so my purpose here is not to replicate those books. Rather, I want to provide an overview of the treatment approaches for chronic Lyme disease and OTBDs so that you understand what is needed to successfully treat these illnesses.

I have encountered people who believe that antibiotics are the sole treatment for chronic Lyme disease. However, I have also encountered people who are afraid of the side effects of antibiotics and focus only on naturopathic treatment. In my personal experience and based on my research (including comments from many, many chronic Lyme patients), my treatment for chronic Lyme disease and tick-borne coinfections has required antibiotics (and other prescription medications) along with naturopathic treatments, including herbal medicines. This is the approach that my Lyme-literate medical doctor is using to treat me, and most other Lyme-literate doctors seem to promote the same.

The combination of antibiotics (and other prescription medications, as needed) along with herbal medicines is, in my view, an approach that balances killing the bacteria with reducing systemic inflammation, boosting the immune system and helping the body heal so that it can better metabolize medications that are used in treatment. Truly healing from chronic Lyme disease (and other coinfections) requires a multipronged approach that treats different organ systems simultaneously but also from multiple perspectives.

Many, if not most, Lyme-literate doctors treat the whole body and the underlying illness (not just the symptoms), and they do it using individualized therapies. Medical clinics that specialize in Lyme treatment often describe their clinics as integrative and functional. This approach is critical to the successful treatment of Lyme and OTBDs; however, the broader medical community in North America is not supportive of integrative and functional medicine. In some jurisdictions, medical licensing boards are actively attempting to make integrative medicine illegal, which would prevent doctors from treating patients with Lyme and OTBDs and make it even more difficult for patients to access adequate treatment.

In treating chronic Lyme disease, there is no one-size-fits-all approach. Antibiotics and/or herbal medicines that work for one person might not work as well for the next. There are many factors that determine why one treatment works or doesn't. For example, the extent of immune dysfunction and systemic inflammation is generally a function of how long a patient has had chronic Lyme disease. Some people are ill for years before a doctor suspects Lyme disease and begins treatment. The longer someone has had chronic Lyme, the more damage has been done and the harder it is to heal from those years of damage.

Because each patient is different, you must be open to trying different medications and approaches and be willing to adjust your treatment approach on the fly. If a medication or herb isn't working, then try others. One of the most important things to keep in mind when treating chronic Lyme disease is that this is a marathon, not a sprint. For example, I am over a year into my treatment and still have at least another year to go. There is no real way to know how long it will take you to heal. So instead of focusing on how long

```
A Reminder

I am not a medical doctor, and I am not prescribing treatment in this
section. I am only sharing my own experience and the information
I have gleaned over the course of my own treatment and reading.
As I mentioned earlier, every Lyme patient is different and will need
different treatment. Consult a Lyme-literate doctor to help you.
```

treatment will take, focus on how you feel and on the increasing number of good days that you have. This is your measure of success.

Although I will focus on medicinal treatments below, understand that treatment isn't limited to medicines. Treatment must also include restorative sleep, reduced stress, exercise, a healthy diet and good mental health. All of these things are critical to regaining your health.

KILLING THE INFECTION

Antibiotics are generally necessary for killing Lyme bacteria (and some tick-borne microbes), but their success will depend in part on what stage of the infection you are in. Antibiotics aren't the only thing that can kill Lyme bacteria; there are herbal medicines that also function this way. However, for those who have suffered from chronic Lyme (and possibly coinfections) for years, antibiotics are often needed to kill the infections.

The conventional wisdom seems to be that antibiotics are important in treating acute (early-stage) Lyme disease. There is about a two-week window of time after a tick bite in which Lyme disease can generally be effectively treated with a sufficient course of antibiotics. They are also necessary for treating most cases of chronic Lyme disease when symptoms are severe, such as those involving the heart (Lyme carditis), the brain (severe neurological effects) or joints (Lyme arthritis). Antibiotics are very important in treating other tick-borne bacterial infections as well, such as bartonellosis, ehrlichiosis, anaplasmosis and RMSF, which can be very dangerous and even fatal.

There are, however, patients who don't get well despite antibiotic treatment. Remember that *Borrelia* bacteria remain in the bloodstream for a relatively short period of time. They disseminate to tissues throughout the body and can form cyst-like round bodies within the tissues where antibiotics can't reach them. They can also form biofilms that protect them from the antibiotics. Antibiotics used for too long or at too high a dose can also kill the good bacteria in the body, especially in the gut, which can result in damage to your immune system. The beneficial microbes in the gut help support immune function, brain function and many other aspects of good health, so you have to find a balance between effective treatment without wiping out all of those good bacteria and opening the door for harmful bacteria to take over. If gut issues become a big problem while taking oral antibiotics, then intravenous delivery or intramuscular injection of antibiotics can be done.

Prescription Drugs
Doxycycline and its relative minocycline are the most commonly prescribed antibiotics for treating Lyme disease. However, a number of different antibiotics can also be used. Research done in

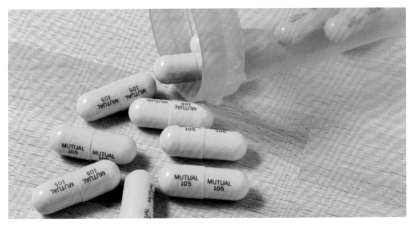

Doxycycline is an antibiotic commonly prescribed in the treatment of Lyme.

Dr. Ying Zhang's lab at Johns Hopkins University tested different antibiotics alone and in combinations, and it found that a combination of three antibiotics — daptomycin, doxycycline and ceftriaxone — was effective at killing *Borrelia* in laboratory studies, and that each one on its own or paired with another was not sufficient to kill the bacteria (Feng et al. 2019). I have since heard some Lyme-literate doctors say that although this combination of three antibiotics was effective at killing *Borrelia* in lab experiments, in practice with Lyme patients, this approach is not as effective. However, clinical studies (along with anecdotal evidence from Lyme-literate doctors who treat thousands of patients) are needed to fully understand the efficacy of Zhang's drug combination for treatment of chronic Lyme.

Another antibiotic that has received more recent attention is dapsone. This antibiotic is known to kill the persister form of *Borrelia* (Horowitz and Freeman 2016). Dapsone can have severe side effects, such as extreme anemia, and so a Lyme-literate doctor should be consulted prior to starting a course of dapsone.

If antibiotics aren't able to kill the *Borrelia* bacteria once they have disseminated and burrowed into various tissues around the body, then what can kill them? In the past few years, a number of Lyme-literate doctors have been using disulfiram, a drug that was historically given to treat alcoholism. Research has shown that in lab studies disulfiram was effective at killing the persister form of *Borrelia* (Alvarez-Manzo et al. 2020). Several well-known Lyme-literate doctors in the United States have also said that they've used disulfiram with success in treating chronic Lyme disease. Disulfiram does have side effects, and alcohol cannot be consumed when taking the medication. A Lyme-literate doctor should be consulted before starting a course of disulfuram.

Herbal Medicines

Herbal medicines are a large and important component for treating chronic Lyme disease and OTBDs. What should be noted

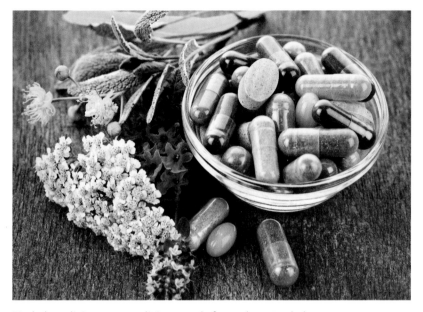

Herbal medicines are medicines made from plants and plant extracts.

is that herbal medicines are just that — medicines. They contain chemical compounds that have medicinal benefits as well as side effects. What makes them different from prescription drugs is that most prescription drugs are either purified or synthesized, making them very potent. Plants contain secondary compounds, which they manufacture often to protect them from being eaten by herbivorous animals. Those secondary compounds are the things that often have medicinal qualities.

Compared to synthetic drugs, herbal medicines generally contain low doses of these compounds, which is why they are often taken over a longer period of time. Also, herbal medicines can have synergistic effects, meaning that they can interact with other herbal medicines in ways that make them more effective than when they are taken on their own. However, you also need to be careful because some medicines interact in harmful ways. This is why a Lyme-literate doctor or naturopath should be consulted when you're deciding which herbal medicines to take.

What Lyme Treatment Can Look Like

These tables show you my list of medications when I first started treatment with my Lyme-literate doctor. Note that this list is only meant to illustrate a treatment plan, and it should not be used as guidance for treating your own Lyme or OTBDs. You should consult a Lyme-literate doctor for your own treatment plan.

Medicine	Treatment Purpose
Azithromycin	Treats babesiosis
Malarone (anti-malarial)	Treats babesiosis
Cryptolepis	Treats babesiosis
Minocycline	Treats Lyme
Fluconazole	Treats mold
Ketoconazole (nasal spray)	Treats mold
BEG Nasal Spray	Treats mold
Nystatin	Treats mold
Low-dose naltrexone	Treats autoimmune dysfunction
Boluoke	Treats Lyme
Artemisinin	Treats Lyme
Biocidin	Busts Lyme biofilms
Kolorex	Treats *Candida*/mold
Saccharomyces boulardii	Acts as binder for removing mycotoxins
Cholestyramine	Acts as binder for removing mycotoxins
Bentonite	Acts as binder for removing mycotoxins
Chlorella	Acts as binder for removing mycotoxins

Medicine	Treatment Purpose
Activated charcoal	Acts as binder for removing mycotoxins
Humic-Monolaurin Complex	Treats autoimmune dysfunction
Cytoquel	Reduces inflammation
Transfer Factor Enviro	Reduces inflammation
GI support supplement	Promotes gut health and helps with leaky gut
Magnesium	Helps with muscle twitching and poor sleep
Vitamins D and K	Gives nutrient support and boosts the immune system
MCT oil	Helps get the body into ketosis
Electrolytes	Helps with muscle twitching and provides electrolytes lost through a keto diet (diuretic diet)

Additional Treatments Added Later	
Medicine	**Treatment Purpose**
Cat's claw	Treats Lyme
Ashwaganda (adaptaogen)	Helps with fatigue, acts as an immune booster and balances hormones
Resveratrol	Reduces inflammation and acts as an antioxidant
N-acetyl cysteine	Reduces inflammation
Zinc	Supports thyroid function
Selenium	Supports thyroid function
B vitamins	Boosts immune function
Liposomal glutathione	Assists with detoxification

I am currently taking upwards of 20 herbal medicines for treatment of my chronic Lyme. It sounds alarming, but when you consider that each one of these serves a function and that together they can have synergistic effects, this number of herbal medicines isn't such a big deal. My biggest challenge is what I call pill fatigue. I'm not a fan of taking pills, and having to swallow a lot of pills each day can be very challenging for me. Some days I just can't do it and miss a dose, which is not good, but I do the best I can. While most of my herbal medicines are in pill form, thankfully some of the remedies I take are powders that I can dissolve in water and drink.

Herbal medicines serve various functions. Some are antimicrobial, meaning that they can kill bacteria and other microbes, such as protozoans, fungi and viruses. Some have anti-inflammatory properties, while others help to boost the immune system. Others have antioxidant properties, help build resistance to stress, help the body to detoxify or help to balance hormones.

CBD

Another plant-derived treatment that helps with body pain, inflammation and sleep disturbance is cannabidiol (CBD), from the cannibis plant. CBD is not psychoactive, so you will not get high from it. It has minimal side effects and can significantly help with Lyme and OTBD symptoms. I have recently started using it, and I find it helps considerably with body pain and sleep. The best approach is to titrate your dosage — meaning start with the smallest dose and increase until you obtain the relief you need. Do this in consultation with a licensed doctor who can monitor you and ensure you are taking an appropriate dose.

Common Treatment Protocols

There are many different treatment protocols for Lyme disease and OTBDs. Before starting any treatment, you should seek the help of a Lyme-literate doctor or naturopath. Here are a few of the widely known treatment protocols that Lyme patients use:

Buhner Protocol: Stephen H. Buhner's treatment protocol is one of the best-known herbal medicine protocols for treating Lyme disease and coinfections.
- *Healing Lyme: Natural Healing and Prevention of Lyme Borreliosis and the Coinfections Chlamydia and Spotted Fever Rickettsiosis*, 2nd edition (2015)
- *Healing Lyme Disease Coinfections: Complementary and Holistic Treatments for Bartonella and Mycoplasma* (2013)

Ross Protocol: Dr. Marty Ross has a treatment protocol that can be downloaded from his website as a free pdf book (treatlyme.net/lyme-disease-treatment-guidelines). He also has excellent videos on his website where he discusses various treatment options and there are links to his book.
- *Antigerm Action Plans for Lyme Disease: How to Use Herbal & Prescription Germ Killers for Bacteria, Parasites, Viruses & Yeast* (2018)

Horowitz Action Plan: Dr. Richard Horowitz's book goes into lots of detail of treatments for various aspects of Lyme disease such as killing the infections, dealing with immune dysfunction and inflammation, environmental toxins, mitochondrial dysfunction and so on.
- *How Can I Get Better? An Action Plan for Treating Resistant Lyme and Chronic Disease* (2017)

Burrascano Treatment Guidelines – Dr. Joseph Burrascano has a free guide about Lyme disease and coinfections, including treatment, which can be downloaded for free (researchednutritionals.com/wp-content/uploads/2016/04/Burrascanos-Advanced-Topics-in-Lyme-Disease-_12_17_08.pdf). He coauthored a book with Dr. Daniel Kinderlehrer.
- *Recovery from Lyme Disease: The Integrative Medicine Guide to Diagnosing and Treating Tick-Borne Illness* (2021)

Rawls Treatment Guidelines: Dr. Bill Rawl's excellent book dives into every aspect of how Lyme and OTBDs affect the body and how to treat it. He also has good resources on his website (rawlsmd.com).
- *Unlocking Lyme: Myths, Truths & Practical Solutions for Chronic Lyme Disease* (2017)

Herxing

Treatments that involve the killing of tick-borne infections can result in something called *herxing*, or experiencing a Jarisch–Herxheimer reaction. During treatment, the body can become overwhelmed by the effects of the dying microbes. This die-off results in the release of cytokines and toxins, which cause inflammation. While herxing, a person's symptoms temporarily worsen before they get better. This can be really hard to deal with when you already feel lousy from the infections you are fighting. In some cases, herxing can get so bad that either the treatment dosage needs to be reduced or, in some cases, it has to be stopped temporarily. Some herxing is typical with Lyme treatment, but there is no point in making yourself really sick just from the treatment, which could actually delay your recovery.

When the medicines you are taking cause infection-causing microbes to die off, cytokines and toxins released during the process can accumulate in your body. Medicines (both prescription and herbal) can act as binders to help remove toxins (including mycotoxins) from the body, but using binders can also induce herxing. Common binders include charcoal caplets, bentonite clay, *Chlorella* (a type of green alga) and cholestyramine (a prescription drug usually used to decrease cholesterol levels in the blood). If you're herxing while using these medicines, talk to your doctor or naturopath about adjusting your dosage to a point where the herxing is tolerable.

OTHER TREATMENTS

Diet is an important part of the treatment of Lyme disease and OTBDs. A healthy diet will help boost your immune system and lower systemic inflammation. Given that leaky gut is often a part of the multisystem effects caused by the *Borrelia* bacteria, eating a gut-friendly diet is critical.

As mentioned earlier, food intolerances can develop as a result of leaky gut; therefore, pay attention to any foods that cause

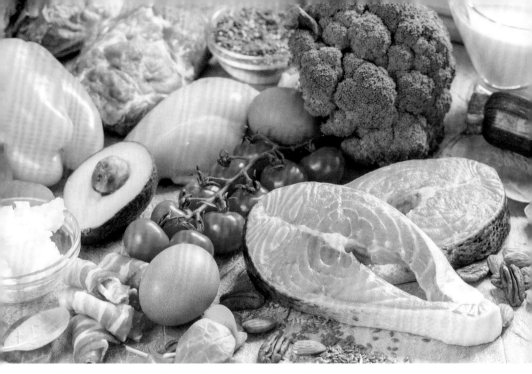

A keto diet — high in fat, moderate in protein and low in carbs — can help stem inflammation and boost your immune system.

discomfort and avoid them. Because one goal of treatment is to reduce systemic inflammation, a specific diet that reduces inflammation is a good idea. Many Lyme patients opt to shift to the ketogenic (keto) diet, a diet that is high in fat, moderate in protein and low in carbohydrates. The diet shifts the body from burning carbohydrates for energy to using fats as the main energy source. You're encouraged to drink plenty of fluids while on a keto diet because the diet has a diuretic effect.

The keto diet is considered by many to be a low-inflammation diet (especially the dairy-free version). It is also beneficial because Lyme bacteria and other microbes depend on carbohydrates to fuel their metabolism, so switching to a keto diet is a way to starve the microbes while also reducing inflammation.

Part of my keto diet involves intermittent fasting. I fast for 16 hours per day, eat only two meals per day, and ensure that I eat those meals within a six- to eight-hour period. Occasionally, I extend my fasting to 18 hours, and now and again I try to go 24 hours without eating. Fasting not only promotes ketosis (the burning of fat as the body's energy source), it also helps to reduce inflammation.

If you are going to shift to a keto diet, consult your Lyme-literate doctor in advance and do your homework to understand how ketosis works, how to stay in ketosis and what foods you can and cannot eat. The dairy-free version of keto (often referred to as paleo keto) is thought to be the best for those with chronic tick-borne infections because dairy (made from cow's milk) can cause inflammation. The challenge I have with paleo keto is getting enough fat in my diet while omitting dairy. There are foods like avocados, which are high in fat, that can help replace dairy; however, I have personally chosen not to eat avocados due to the environmental and social impacts of the avocado industry. What you are willing to buy and eat are personal choices that you need to make for yourself.

In addition to antibiotics and other prescription drugs, herbal medicines and diet, there are numerous other treatments. Some are solidly based on science, whereas others, to me, seem less so. Detailing these other treatments is far beyond the scope of this book, but I encourage you to consult a Lyme-literate doctor to discuss the range of treatment options.

The bottom line in treating chronic Lyme disease and OTBDs is that it is a long process. There will be setbacks, times when you feel you are not progressing in your healing and you may even feel as if you are going backward. Unfortunately, this is a normal part of the battle with Lyme. The process of healing can also be expensive, sometimes costing thousands to hundreds of thousands of dollars. In some cases chronic Lyme disease can be cured, while for other people, remission may be the best outcome they can hope for. The goal then becomes to remain in remission as long as possible and to use medicines, diet and other approaches to manage flare-ups.

Conclusion

As this book has demonstrated, Lyme disease is a very complex disease caused by a bacterial infection that can do serious harm to your health if not treated adequately. Chronic Lyme and OTBDs can be very difficult to eradicate, and some people may never fully recover, though remission with occasional flare-ups seems to be achievable by many. It's scary to think that something like a casual hike in the woods could lead to months and even years of debilitating illness, and it can be disheartening to realize that every stage of this disease — from diagnosis to treatment to, hopefully, recovery — is a marathon, not a sprint, and the road to recovery is a steep, uphill one. Ultimately, this is a road you *can* travel successfully. Mindset matters. As with any illness, it is important to remain optimistic about recovery and not feel discouraged about setbacks. Treatment for Lyme and OTBDs requires individualized care, so if a treatment isn't working for you, talk to your Lyme-literate doctor about trying something else. Above all, don't give up!

There is a lot of information in this book for you to digest and understand. However, here are some key take-home messages for you to keep in mind as you navigate your journey with Lyme and OTBDs:

- You don't have to face your battle with Lyme and OTBDs alone. Lean on those close to you for support. I also recommend that you use the Internet to locate a Lyme support group near you. There are also many Lyme support groups on Facebook. Empathy can play an important role in getting you through the tough times. The only people who will truly know what you're going through are those who are going through it or have gone through it. Reach out to them for help.
- Find a Lyme-literate medical doctor who will create a person-alized treatment plan tailored to your specific symptoms and infections and who will offer you the option of being treated

under ILADS guidelines. Most Lyme-literate doctors use a functional, integrative approach to treating the causes of the illness and not just the symptoms.

- Take it one day at a time. Be sure to adjust your expectations, at least temporarily. I have always been a high-energy person, doing 20 things at once. I have a passion for life and never do anything by half measure. However, with my Lyme disease and OTBDs, I've had to greatly reduce my workload and the stress in my life. I've learned that I must take more time to relax, rest and care for myself, and I must put my health before anything else. Be kind to yourself, and when you feel you need a rest or just don't have the energy to complete a task, accept it and don't beat yourself up about it.
- If you're worried about being infected or reinfected with a tick-borne disease, remember that hiding indoors isn't the solution. Being in nature offers so many rewards both to your mental and physical health. As you read in Chapter 3, there are several effective measures you can take to reduce the risk of a tick bite without reducing your enjoyment of the outdoors.

What does the future hold for those suffering from Lyme and OTBDs? Where is the science of tick-borne diseases headed? And what changes do we need to see in the diagnosis and treatment of Lyme and OTBDs?

First and foremost, we need respect for patients to be restored. It is alarmingly common for patients with Lyme and/or OTBDs to be belittled, berated, insulted, ignored and denied treatment by primary care doctors because of the diseases those patients were unfortunate enough to contract. No person, regardless of the disease or ailment they have, deserves to be treated poorly. The scientific body of evidence for the existence of chronic Lyme is substantial. Primary care doctors need to stop looking solely to the IDSA Guidelines and, instead, look to peer-reviewed scientific literature, which widely acknowledges the existence of chronic Lyme. Until the denial of chronic Lyme ends, many more people will suffer needlessly, and the financial burden of chronic illness on both individuals and our health care systems will continue to grow.

Of course, this body of scientific research around Lyme disease and OTBDs is still growing and gaining momentum. Research on treatment options, especially using herbal medicines, is receiving more attention than ever. However, additional properly controlled clinical studies are still needed to further develop effective treatment options and bolster the toolkit of medicines available for the treatment of Lyme, especially the persister forms of Lyme, which are so hard to eradicate.

Lyme and OTBDs have put our medical systems to the test — systems that, more often than not, are failing thousands of patients who need help and compassion desperately. Lyme and OTBDs are also challenging our understanding of how the human immune system works. In particular, there is a growing body of evidence supporting the idea that diseases such as MS, ALS, lupus, Parkinson's and Alzheimer's have a basis in immune dysfunction and that this may, in at least some cases, be caused by an infectious agent (like a bacterium, virus, fungus or parasite). Research into PANDAS (pediatric autoimmune neuropsychiatric disorder associated with Streptococcus) and PANS (pediatric acute-onset neuropsychiatric syndrome) is paving the way to understanding how infection can produce abnormal activation of the immune system, leading to extreme neuropsychiatric problems, especially in children.

Other research also shows evidence that some people may be genetically more susceptible to infections and may produce inappropriate or inadequate immune responses to infectious agents. Could this shed light on chronic Lyme sufferers? Approximately 20 percent of Lyme patients go on to develop chronic Lyme disease, a statistic commonly found in Lyme literature. Is it possible that these 20 percent belong to a subpopulation with a genetic makeup that predisposes them to immune dysfunction in response to infectious agents and environmental toxins? New research is generating gene theories like the RCCX Theory, which suggests that mutations in this gene region may cause autoimmune and inflammatory disorders that may result in diseases such as chronic fatigue, Epstein-Barr infection, mold toxicity, psychiatric conditions and Lyme disease. Research funding needs to be directed at testing ideas like these that may help us understand the basis of these illnesses.

If the medical profession acknowledges and accepts the growing body of peer-reviewed research on Lyme and OTBDs, then one day we may truly understand the science of these diseases and be able to finally help those who so desperately need adequate medical care. To get there will require collaboration between medical researchers, primary care doctors, other health professionals, patients and government policy makers. Working together will not only lead to the development of more effective diagnostic tools and treatments but also bridge a divide that is currently causing immeasurable pain and suffering for patients dealing with Lyme and OTBDs. I am hopeful that these challenges can be overcome and lead to a better future for those suffering from Lyme and OTBDs.

BIBLIOGRAPHY

Alvarez-Manzo, Hector S., Yumin Zhang, Wanliang Shi and Ying Zhang. "Evaluation of Disulfiram Drug Combinations and Identification of Other More Effective Combinations Against Stationary Phase *Borrelia burgdorferi*." *Antibiotics (Basel)* 9, no. 9 (August 2020): 542–556.

Anderson, J.F., R.C. Johnson, L.A. Magnarelli and F.W. Hyde. "Involvement of Birds in the Epidemiology of the Lyme Disease Agent *Borrelia burgdorferi*." *Infection and Immunity* 51, no. 2 (February 1986): 394–396.

Binetruy, Florian, Stéphane Garnier, Nathalie Boulanger, Émilie Talagrand-Reboul, Etienne Loire, Bruno Faivre, Valérie Noël, Marie Buysse and Olivier Duron. "A Novel *Borrelia* Species, Intermediate Between Lyme Disease and Relapsing Fever Groups, in Neotropical Passerine-Associated Ticks." *Scientific Reports* 10, article no. 10596 (June 2020).

Bowman, A.S. and J.R. Sauer. "Tick Salivary Glands: Function, Physiology and Future." *Parasitology* 129, S1 (2004): S67–S81.

Buhner, Stephen Harrod. *Healing Lyme: Natural Healing and Prevention of Lyme Borreliosis and Its Coinfections*. Raven Press, 2005.

Bui-Klimke, Travis R. and Felicia Wu. "Ochratoxin A and Human Health Risk: A Review of the Evidence." *Critical Reviews in Food Science and Nutrition* 55, no. 13 (2015): 1860–1869.

Cameron, Daniel J., Lorraine B. Johnson and Elizabeth L. Maloney. "Evidence Assessments and Guideline Recommendations in Lyme Disease: The Clinical Management of Known Tick Bites, Erythema Migrans Rashes and Persistent Disease." *Expert Review of Anti-Infective Therapy* 12, no. 9 (September 2014): 1103–1135.

Canadian Public Health Laboratory Network (CPHLN) "The Laboratory Diagnosis of Lyme Borreliosis: Guidelines from the Canadian Public Health Laboratory Network." *The Canadian Journal of Infectious Diseases and Medical Microbiology* 18, no. 2 (March 2007): 145–148.

Cassarino, David S., Martha M. Quezado, Nitya R. Ghatak and Paul H. Duray. "Lyme-Associated Parkinsonism: A Neuropathologic Case Study and Review of the Literature." *Archives of Pathology and Laboratory Medicine* 127, no. 9 (September 2003): 1204–1206.

Centers for Disease Control and Prevention. "Recommendations for Test Performance and Interpretation from Second National Conference on Serologic Diagnosis of Lyme Disease." *Morbidity and Mortality Weekly Report* 44 (1995): 590–591.

Chmielewska-Badora J., E. Cisak and J. Dutkiewicz. "Lyme Borreliosis and Multiple Sclerosis: Any Connection? A Seroepidemic Study." *Annals of Agricultural and Environmental Medicine* 7, no. 2 (February 2000): 141–143.

Clow, K.M. "The Ecology and Epidemiology of the Blacklegged Tick, *Ixodes scapularis*, and the Risk of Lyme Disease in Ontario, Canada." Doctoral thesis, University of Guelph, 2017.

Cook, Michael J. "Lyme Borreliosis: A Review of Data on Transmission Time After Tick Attachment." *International Journal of General Medicine* 19, no. 8 (2015):1–8.

Cook, Michael J. and Basant K. Puri. "Commercial Test Kits for Detection of Lyme Borreliosis: A Meta-Analysis of Test Accuracy." *International Journal of General Medicine* 18, no. 9 (2016): 427–440.

Cutler, Sally J., Eva Ruzic-Sabljic and Aleksandar Potkonjak. "Emerging *Borreliae* – Expanding Beyond Lyme Borreliosis." *Molecular and Cellular Probes* 31 (February 2017): 22–27.

Edlow, Jonathan A. *Bull's Eye: Unraveling the Medical Mystery of Lyme Disease.* New Haven: Yale University Press, 2003.

Evason, Michelle, Jason W. Stull, David L. Pearl, Andrew S. Peregrine, Claire Jardine, Jesse S. Buch, Zachary Lailer, Tom O'Connor, Ramaswamy Chandrashekar and J. Scott Weese. "Prevalence of *Borrelia burgdorferi*, *Anaplasma* spp., *Ehrlichia* spp. and *Dirofilaria immitis* in Canadian Dogs, 2008 to 2015: A Repeat Cross-Sectional Study." *Parasites & Vectors* 12, no. 1 (January 2019): 64.

Feng, Jie, Tingting Li, Rebecca Yee, Yuting Yuan, Chunxiang Bai, Menghua Cai, Wanliang Shi, Monica Embers, Cory Brayton, Harumi Saeki, Kathleen Gabrielson and Ying Zhang. "Stationary Phase Persister/Biofilm Microcolony of *Borrelia burgdorferi* Causes More Severe Disease in a Mouse Model of Lyme Arthritis: Implications for Understanding Persistence, Post-Treatment Lyme Disease Syndrome (PTLDS), and Treatment Failure." *Discovery Medicine* 27, no. 148 (March 2019): 125–138.

Francischetti, Ivo M.B., Anderson Sá-Nunes, Ben J. Mans, Isabel M. Santos and José M.C. Ribeiro. "The Role of Saliva in Tick Feeding." *Frontiers of Bioscience* 14 (January 2009): 2051–2088.

Fritzsche, Markus. "Chronic Lyme Borreliosis at the Root of Multiple Sclerosis -- Is a Cure with Antibiotics Attainable?" *Medical Hypotheses* 64, no. 3 (2005): 438–448.

Horowitz, Richard I. *Why Can't I Get Better? Solving the Mystery of Lyme and Chronic Disease.* St. Martin's Press, 2013.

Horowitz, Richard I. and Phyllis R. Freeman. "The Use of Dapsone as a Novel 'Persister' Drug in the Treatment of Chronic Lyme Disease/Post Treatment Lyme Disease Syndrome." *Journal of Clinical & Experimental Dermatology Research* 7, no. 3 (January 2016).

Jarefors, Sara, Louise Bennet, Elin You, Pia Forsberg, Christina Ekerfelt, Johan Berglund and Jan Ernerudh. "Lyme Borreliosis Reinfection: Might It Be Explained by a Gender Difference in Immune Response?" *Immunology* 118, no. 2 (June 2006): 224–232.

Keller, Andreas, Angela Graefen, Markus Ball, Mark Matzas, Valesca Boisguerin, Frank Maixner, Petra Leidinger, Christina Backes, Rabab Khairat, Michael Forster, Björn Stade, Andre Franke, Jens Mayer, Jessica Spangler, Stephen McLaughlin, Minita Shah, Clarence Lee, Timothy T. Harkins, Alexander Sartori, Andres Moreno-Estrada, Brenna Henn, Martin Sikora, Ornella Semino, Jacques Chiaroni, Siiri Rootsi, Natalie M. Myres, Vicente M. Cabrera, Peter A. Underhill, Carlos D. Bustamante, Eduard Egarter Vigl, Marco Samadelli, Giovanna Cipollini, Jan Haas, Hugo Katus, Brian D. O'Connor, Marc R.J. Carlson, Benjamin Meder, Nikolaus Blin, Eckart Meese, Carsten M. Pusch and Albert Zink. "New Insights into the Tyrolean Iceman's Origin and Phenotype as Inferred by Whole-Genome Sequencing." *Nature Communications* 3 (February 2012): 698.

LaFleur, Rhonda L., Steven M. Callister, Jennifer C. Dant, Dean A. Jobe, Steven D. Lovrich, Thomas F. Warner, Terri L. Wasmoen and Ronald F. Schell. "One-Year Duration of Immunity Induced by Vaccination with a Canine Lyme Disease Bacterin." *Clinical and Vaccine Immunology* 17, no. 5 (May 2010): 870–874.

Lantos P.M., J. Rumbaugh, L.K. Bockenstedt et al. "Clinical Practice Guidelines by the Infectious Diseases Society of America, American Academy of Neurology, and American College of Rheumatology: 2020 Guidelines for the Prevention, Diagnosis, and Treatment of Lyme Disease." *Neurology* 96, no. 6 (February 2021): 262–273.

Liang, Liucun, Jinyong Wang, Lucas Schorter, Thu Phong Nguyen Trong, Shari Fell, Sebastian Ulrich and Reinhard K. Straubinger. "Rapid Clearance of *Borrelia burgdorferi* from the Blood Circulation." *Parasites & Vectors* 13, article no. 191 (April 2020).

Lloyd, Vett K. and Ralph G. Hawkins. "Under-Detection of Lyme Disease in Canada." *Healthcare (Basel)* 6, no. 4 (October 2018): 125

Marsh, P.D. "Dental Plaque as a Microbial Biofilm." *Caries Research* 38, no. 3 (May–June 2004): 204–211.

Meriläinen, Leena, Anni Herranen, Armin Schwarzbach and Leona Gilbert. "Morphological and Biochemical Features of *Borrelia burgdorferi* Pleomorphic Forms." *Microbiology* 161, no. 3 (March 2015): 516–527.

Middelveen, Marianne J., Jennie Burke, Eva Sapi, Cheryl Bandoski, Katherine R. Filush, Yean Wang, Agustin Franco, Arun Timmaraju, Hilary A. Schlinger, Peter J. Mayne and Raphael B. Stricker. "Culture and Identification of *Borrelia* Spirochetes in Human Vaginal and Seminal Secretions." *F1000 Research* 3 (December 2014): 309.

Nathan, Neil. *Toxic: Heal Your Body from Mold Toxicity, Lyme Disease, Multiple Chemical Sensitivities, and Chronic Environmental Illness*. Victory Belt Publishing Inc., 2018.

Nelder, Mark P., Curtis B. Russell, Steven Johnson, Ye Li, Kirby Cronin, Bryna Warshawsky, Nicolas Brandon and Samir N. Patel. "Assessing Human Exposure to Spotted Fever and Typhus Group *Rickettsiae* in Ontario, Canada (2013–2018): A Retrospective, Cross-Sectional Study." *BMC Infectious Diseases* 20, article no. 523 (July 2020).

Pfeiffer, Mary Beth. *Lyme: The First Epidemic of Climate Change*. Island Press, 2018

Pisché, Guillaume, Meriam Koob, Thomas Wirth, Véronique Quenardelle, Ouhaïd Lagha-Boukbiza, Mathilde Renaud, Mathieu Anheim and Christine Tranchant. "Subacute Parkinsonism as a Complication of Lyme Disease." *Journal of Neurology* 264, no. 5 (May 2017): 1015–1019.

Poinar, George, Jr. "Spirochete-Like Cells in a Dominican Amber *Amblyomma* Tick (Arachnida: Ixodidae)." *An International Journal of Paleobiology* 27, no. 5 (2015): 565–570.

Rauter, Carolin, Markus Mueller, Isabel Diterich, Sabine Zeller, Dieter Hassler, Thomas Meergans and Thomas Hartung. "Critical Evaluation of Urine-Based PCR Assay for Diagnosis of Lyme Borreliosis." *Clinical and Diagnostic Laboratory Immunology* 12, no. 8 (August 2005): 910–917.

Rawls, William. *Unlocking Lyme: Myths, Truths, and Practical Solutions for Chronic Lyme Disease*. FirstDoNoHarm Publishing, 2017.

Rebman, Alison W., Mark J. Soloski, and John N. Aucott. "Sex and Gender Impact Lyme Disease Immunopathology, Diagnosis and Treatment." In *Sex and Gender Differences in Infection and Treatments for Infectious Diseases*, edited by S. Klein and C. Roberts, 337–360. Springer International Publishing, 2015.

Rudenko, Nataliia, Maryna Golovchenko, Libor Grubhoffer and James H. Oliver Jr. "Updates on *Borrelia burgdorferi sensu lato* Complex with Respect to Public Health." *Ticks and Tick-Borne Diseases* 2, no. 3 (September 2011): 123–128.

Sapi, Eva, Rumanah S. Kasliwala, Hebo Ismail, Jason P. Torres, Michael Oldakowski, Sarah Markland, Gauri Gaur, Anthony Melillo, Klaus Eisendle, Kenneth B. Liegner, Jenny Libien and James E. Goldman. "The Long-Term Persistence of *Borrelia burgdorferi* Antigens and DNA in the Tissues of a Patient with Lyme Disease." *Antibiotics (Basel)* 8, no. 4 (October 2019): 183.

Schaller, James. *The Diagnosis and Treatment of Babesia: Lyme's Cruel Cousin -- The Other Tick-Borne Infection*. Hope Academic Press, 2006.

Scheffold, Norbert, Bernhard Herkommer, Reinhard Kandolf and Andreas E. May. "Lyme Carditis -- Diagnosis, Treatment and Prognosis." *Deutsches Ärzteblatt International* 112, no. 12 (March 2015): 202–208.

Scherler, Aurélie, Nicolas Jacquier and Gilbert Greub. "*Chlamydiales, Anaplasma* and *Bartonella*: Persistence and Immune Escape of Intracellular Bacteria." *Microbes and Infection* 20, nos. 7–8 (August–September 2018): 416–423.

Schöllkopf, Claudia, Mads Melbye, Lars Munksgaard, Karin Ekström Smedby, Klaus Rostgaard, Bengt Glimelius, Ellen T. Chang, Göran Roos, Mads Hansen, Hans-Olov Adami and Henrik Hjalgrim. "*Borrelia* Infection and Risk of Non-Hodgkin Lymphoma." *Blood* 111, no. 12 (June 2008): 5524–5529.

Schwarzwalder, Alison, Michael F. Schneider, Alison Lydecker, John N. Aucott. "Sex Differences in the Clinical and Serologic Presentation of Early Lyme Disease: Results from a Retrospective Review." *Gender Medicine* 7, no. 4 (August 2010): 320–329.

Scott, John D. and Lance A. Durden. "New Records of the Lyme Disease Bacterium in Ticks Collected from Songbirds in Central and Eastern Canada." *International Journal of Acarology* 41, no. 4 (2015): 241–249.

Sertour, Natacha, Violaine Cotté, Martine Garnier, Laurence Malandrin, Elisabeth Ferquel and Valérie Choumet. "Infection Kinetics and Tropism of *Borrelia burgdorferi sensu lato* in Mouse after Natural (via Ticks) or Artificial (Needle) Infection Depends on the Bacterial Strain." *Frontiers in Microbiology* 9, article no. 1722 (July 2018).

Shih, C.M. and A. Spielman. "Accelerated Transmission of Lyme Disease Spirochetes by Partially Fed Vector Ticks." *Journal of Clinical Microbiology* 31, no. 11 (November 1993): 2878–2881.

Stanek, G. and M. Reiter. "The Expanding Lyme *Borrelia* Complex -- Clinical Significance of Genomic Species?" *Clinical Microbiology and Infection* 17, no. 4 (April 2011): 487–493.

Stonehouse, Amber, James S. Studdiford and C. Amber Henry. "An Update on the Diagnosis and Treatment of Early Lyme Disease: Focusing on the Bull's Eye, You May Miss the Mark." *Journal of Emergency Medicine* 39, no. 5 (November 2010): e147–151.

Stricker, Raphael B. and Lorraine Johnson. "Gender Bias in Chronic Lyme Disease." *Journal of Women's Health* 18, no. 10 (October 2009): 1717–1718.

Stricker, Raphael B. and Marianne J. Middelveen. "Sexual Transmission of Lyme Disease: Challenging the Tickborne Disease Paradigm." *Expert Review of Anti-Infective Therapy* 13, no. 11 (2015): 1303–1306.

Stricker, Raphael B., D.H. Moore and E.E. Winger. "Clinical and Immunologic Evidence for Transmission of Lyme Disease through Intimate Human Contact." *Journal of Investigative Medicine* 52, S1 (January 2004): S151.

Tager, Felice A., Brian A. Fallon, John Keilp, Marian Rissenberg, Charles Ray Jones and Michael R. Liebowitz. "A Controlled Study of Cognitive Deficits in Children with Chronic Lyme Disease." *Journal of Neuropsychiatry and Clinical Neurosciences* 13, no. 4 (November 2001): 500–507.

Talkington, Jeffrey and Steven P. Nickell. "*Borrelia burgdorferi* Spirochetes Induce Mast Cell Activation and Cytokine Release." *Infection and Immunity* 67, no. 3 (March 1999): 1107–1115.

Tijsse-Klassen, Ellen, Nenad Pandak, Paul Hengeveld, Katsuhisa Takumi, Marion P.G. Koopmans and Hein Sprong. "Ability to Cause Erythema Migrans Differs Between *Borrelia burgdorferi sensu lato* Isolates." *Parasites & Vectors* 6, article no. 2330 (2013).

Tørnqvist-Johnsen, Camilla, Sara-Ann Dickson, Kerry Rolph, Valentina Palermo, Hannah Hodgkiss-Geere, Paul Gilmore, and Danièlle A. Gunn-Moore. "First Report of Lyme Borreliosis Leading to Cardiac Bradydysrhythmia in Two Cats." *Journal of Feline Medicine and Surgery Open Reports* 6, no. 1 (January 2020).

Yeung, Cynthia and Adrian Baranchuk. "Systematic Approach to the Diagnosis and Treatment of Lyme Carditis and High-Degree Atrioventricular Block." *Healthcare (Basel)* 6, no. 4 (September 2018): 119.

RESOURCES

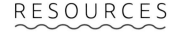

Books

Unlocking Lyme: Myths, Truths & Practical Solutions for Chronic Lyme Disease by William Rawls, MD (2017, FirstDoNoHarm Publishing)

Why Can't I Get Better? Solving the Mystery of Lyme and Chronic Disease by Richard I. Horowitz, MD (2013, St. Martin's Press)

How Can I Get Better? An Action Plan for Treating Resistant Lyme and Chronic Disease by Richard I. Horowitz, MD (2017, St. Martin's Press)

Healing Lyme: Natural Healing and Prevention of Lyme Borreliosis and the Coinfections Chlamydia and Spotted Fever Rickettsioses, 2nd edition, by Stephen Harrod Buhner (2015, Raven Press)

The Top 10 Lyme Disease Treatments: Defeat Lyme Disease with the Best Conventional and Alternative Medicine by Bryan Rosner, foreword by James Schaller, MD (2007, BM Publishing Group)

Toxic: Heal Your Body from Mold Toxicity, Lyme Disease, Multiple Chemical Sensitivities, and Chronic Environmental Illness by Neil Nathan, MD (2018, Victory Belt Publishing Inc.)

The Diagnosis and Treatment of Babesia, Lyme's Cruel Cousin: The Other Tick-Borne Infection by James Schaller, MD (2006, Hope Academic Press)

Lyme Disease: Medical Myopia and the Hidden Global Pandemic by Dr. Bernard Raxlen with Allie Cashel (2019, Hammersmith Books Limited)

Lyme: The First Epidemic of Climate Change by Mary Beth Pfeiffer (2018, Island Press)

The Wahls Protocol: A Radical New Way to Treat All Chronic Autoimmune Conditions Using Paleo Principles by Terry Wahls, MD, with Eve Adamson (2014, Avery)

Websites

CanLyme: canlyme.com
Lyme Disease.org: lymedisease.org
Lyme Ontario: lymeontario.com
Lyme Hope: lymehope.ca
Global Lyme Alliance: globallymealliance.org
Lyme Disease Association: lymediseaseassociation.org
Lyme Disease Foundation: lyme.org
Bay Area Lyme Foundation: bayarealyme.org
International Lyme and Associated Diseases Society (ILADS): ilads.org
Infectious Disease Society of America (IDSA): idsociety.org
    /practice-guideline/lyme-disease
G. Magnotta Foundation: gmagnottafoundation.com/about

Videos

Johns Hopkins Rheumatology, "Think the Lyme Disease Rash is Always a Bull's-eye? Think Again! | Johns Hopkins Rheumatology," uploaded May 7, 2020, Youtube video, 5:50, https://youtu.be/fXLWmtro-ZE

Johns Hopkins Rheumatology, "Understanding the Persistent Symptoms in Lyme Disease | Johns Hopkins Medicine," uploaded May 14, 2020, Youtube video, 8:13, https://youtu.be/EyK-1271xqo

Friends Health Connection, "How to treat resistant lyme disease and chronic disease with Dr. Richard Horowitz," uploaded February 15, 2018, Youtube video, 43:30, https://youtu.be/92pi2R0SYz8

Visit LymeDisease.org, "What natural treatments work for Lyme disease? What are their side effects?," uploaded January 7, 2019, Youtube video, 4:08, https://youtu.be/DisSlelVcrc

LymeMIND, "4th Annual 'Lyme Disease in the Era of Precision Medicine' Conference: Richard Horowitz," uploaded August 28, 2020, Youtube video, 19:54, https://youtu.be/ML-kbOTKAOg

Official W5, "W5: Canadians fight for Lyme disease diagnosis and treatment," uploaded November 21, 2020, Youtube video, 22:21, https://youtu.be/DQh_XPU0imQ

ILADS, "2018 ILADS Webinar - History of Lyme Disease by Joseph J. Burrascano, Jr. MD," uploaded December 17, 2018, Vimeo, 42:30, https://vimeo.com/306846706

VivaPlus Videoproducties, "S.O.S. Lyme, An Invisible Epidemic," uploaded April 9, 2019, Vimeo, 50:23, https://vimeo.com/329276536

Podcasts

Looking at Lyme (by CanLyme): lookingatlyme.ca

Lyme Voice: lymevoice.com/category/podcast

Ticktective (Bay Area Lyme Foundation): bayarealyme.org/video-library/our-podcasts

ACKNOWLEDGMENTS

I wrote this book because I want to help people. I want to help them understand Lyme and OTBDs, recognize what challenges they are up against in getting diagnosis and treatment, and learn "the basics" of Lyme and OTBDs so they can become strong and vocal advocates for themselves or their loved ones. I wouldn't have arrived at writing this book without the many people who have helped me along the way. This book is my way of paying it forward and expressing my gratitude to those who supported and continue to support me and other sufferers through one of the biggest challenges of our lives.

My heartfelt thanks to Dr. Janet Sperling. She was one of the first people I spoke to about the possibility of Lyme disease and coinfections as the source for my illness. She is a wealth of information on the science of Lyme and coinfections as well as a great source of encouragement. Without her help I don't think my recovery to this point would have been possible.

My sincere thanks to my friend Kathy McPherson. Her advice was fundamental to my obtaining a diagnosis and getting started with treatment, and her constant encouragement along the way kept me hopeful. Thank you, Kath.

My deepest thanks to Jennifer Wheeler, a friend and fellow feisty Lyme warrior, whom I cannot thank enough for the reams of information she has shared that have helped me find and fight for my treatment. She has influenced this book in so many ways. She also reviewed a draft of the manuscript in an incredibly short timeframe. I am grateful for the many hours of conversation we have had that have helped to shape my thinking about Lyme and OTBDs. She introduced me to the idea of genetic mutations as an underlying reason for why some people don't get sick from a tick bite while others do. I thank her for her dedication to the battle against Lyme and OTBDs and all that she does in fighting for the rights of Lyme patients. Her energy, commitment, selflessness and dedication are exemplary.

Thanks so much to Julie Cable, Dana Cote, Gerri Foster Norwood and others in my community and beyond who have provided support and advice about treatment. Their help and empathy have been a huge part of my surviving this illness. There were times when I thought these diseases would be the end of me, but thanks to them and others, even on the darkest days, I did not give up.

A very big thank you to those medical professionals who were willing to help me, even in some small way. Sadly, they are few and far between, but those who did help are compassionate people who are dedicated to alleviating suffering. Most especially, I want to thank my current medical team who is overseeing my specialized treatment and recovery. Their knowledge, caring and dedication to providing help to Lyme patients who are otherwise cast aside is phenomenal. I know they are inundated with patients desperate for their expertise, but their tireless work and dedication is so important and so much appreciated. I especially want to thank Jackie F. for her incredible caring, compassion and empathy. I hope she knows how much of a difference she makes to those of us enduring "Lyme Hell." Treating Lyme and OTBDs requires individualized care, which takes a lot of time and effort. It isn't straightforward, and most of the time it feels like trying to hit a moving target. Regardless, Jackie ensures patients receive the best possible individualized care and that we are treated with respect and compassion along the way. ⚠️⚠️⚠️ Jackie.

Lyme disease is a very isolating illness. When it seemed like no doctor would help me, the isolation became worse and I felt like nobody valued my life. And yet, during those darkest days, there were friends who helped me continue to put one foot in front of the other. My sincere thanks to my friend Sandra Shaw for getting me to medical appointments far from home, providing advice and perspective, and her concern and care. And to my longtime friend Donna Pretty, a heartfelt thank you. Empathy is my elixir; thank you for being there for me. A big thanks also to the friends who reached out and asked if I was okay, how I was feeling or if I needed anything. I hope they know how much I appreciate their concern, their kindness and their offers of help. It's amazing how much the words "How are you?" can mean to someone.

Thank you to my fellow CanLyme (Canadian Lyme Disease Foundation) board members for their dedication to creating positive change in the Lyme world. What they do makes a difference.

My heartfelt thanks to the team at Firefly Books: Lionel Koffler, Julie Takasaki, Hartley Millson, Melissa Zilberberg and freelance editor Anne Godlewski. What great people to work with. I am particularly indebted to my editor, Julie Takasaki. Writing this book, while dealing with the isolation of COVID-19 and awful flare-ups of Lyme and OTBD symptoms, has been far more challenging than I thought it would be. Lyme flare-ups pushed deadlines back, but Julie's efficiency and hard work kept us on track. I am so grateful for her compassion and patience and for making this project so much fun.

Finally, to all those around the world who are tireless advocates for those of us with Lyme disease and OTBDs — thank you. It is with your dedication and determination that we will change things for the better. Despite the David and Goliath battle, we will get there.

PHOTO CREDITS

Interior

CDC: 43 (top and bottom), 47, 59, 70, 74, 82 (all except bottom right), 87, 89, 111

CDC/Claudia Molins: 21

CDC/Dr. George R. Healy: 107

CDC/Dr. Sherif Zaki: 90

CDC/James Gathany: 38, 39 (all except Pacific coast tick), 81

George Poinar, Jr., courtesy of Oregon State University (CC BY-SA 2.0): 22

Panther Media GmbH/Alamy Stock Photo: 29

Peter J. Bryant, University of California, Irvine: 39 (Pacific coast tick)

Rocky Mountain Laboratories, National Institutes of Health: 23

Shelley Ball: 8

Shutterstock
Afanasiev Andrii: 72; Aleksei Ruzhin: 20; AmyLv: 55; BalanceFormCreative: 52; Baptiste LEROY - RAWMinet: 45; CGN089: 64; Csaba Deli: 102; dhvstockphoto: 126; Elena Elisseeva: 139; Elena Shashkina: 145; Elizaveta Galitckaia: 56; Fox_Ana: 60; Izf: 68; Jim Cumming: 40; Lordn: 114; Love Lego: 113; macro lens: 32; makasana photo: 103; meunierd: 49; Mironmax Studio: 76; Natalya Erofeeva: 100; Pierre Williot: 50; Prostock-studio: 88; Roman Zaiets: 120; Rudchenko Liliia: 132; Saiful: 123; Sten Roosvald: 67; Steve Hamann: 137; Steven Ellingson: 34; Szasz-Fabian Jozsef: 27; Vovantarakan: 75; Weerapon Nantawisit: 93

Wikimedia Commons/Guswen (CC BY-SA 4.0): 96

Wikimedia Commons/Mikael Häggström: 82 (bottom right)

Back cover

Author photo by Mary Ellen Gucciardi